FOOD AND NU AT RISK IN AMERICA: FOOD INSECURITY, BIOTECHNOLOGY, FOOD SAFETY, AND BIOTERRORISM

Sari Edelstein, PhD, RD
Department of Nutrition
Simmons College

Bonnie L. Gerald, PhD, DTR
Department of Nutrition and Food Systems
University of Southern Mississippi

Tamara M. Crutchley Bushell, PhD
Department of Microbiology
University of Alabama at Birmingham

Craig Gundersen, PhD
Human Development and Family Studies Department
Iowa State University

With Preface by: Alison Harmon, PhD, RD, LN
Health and Human Development
Montana State University

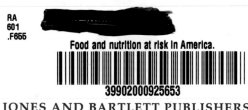

JONES AND BARTLETT PUBLISHERS
Sudbury, Massachusetts
BOSTON   TORONTO   LONDON   SINGAPORE

World Headquarters

Jones and Bartlett Publishers
40 Tall Pine Drive
Sudbury, MA 01776
978-443-5000
info@jbpub.com
www.jbpub.com

Jones and Bartlett Publishers
Canada
6339 Ormindale Way
Mississauga, Ontario L5V 1J2
Canada

Jones and Bartlett Publishers
International
Barb House, Barb Mews
London W6 7PA
United Kingdom

Jones and Bartlett's books and products are available through most bookstores and online booksellers. To contact Jones and Bartlett Publishers directly, call 800-832-0034, fax 978-443-8000, or visit our website www.jbpub.com.

Substantial discounts on bulk quantities of Jones and Bartlett's publications are available to corporations, professional associations, and other qualified organizations. For details and specific discount information, contact the special sales department at Jones and Bartlett via the above contact information or send an email to specialsales@jbpub.com.

This publication is designed to provide accurate and authoritative information in regard to the Subject Matter covered. It is sold with the understanding that the publisher is not engaged in rendering legal, accounting, or other professional service. If legal advice or other expert assistance is required, the service of a competent professional person should be sought.

Production Credits
Publisher: Michael Brown
Production Director: Amy Rose
Associate Editor: Katey Birtcher
Production Editor: Tracey Chapman
Marketing Manager: Sophie Fleck
Manufacturing and Inventory Control
  Supervisor: Amy Bacus

Composition: Auburn Associates, Inc.
Cover Design: Brian Moore
Cover Image: © Matthew Collingwood/
ShutterStock, Inc.; © Elena Elisseeva/
ShutterStock, Inc.; © Kang Khoon
Seang/ShutterStock, Inc.
Printing and Binding: Malloy, Inc.
Cover Printing: Malloy, Inc.

Library of Congress Cataloging-in-Publication Data
Food and nutrition at risk in America: food insecurity, biotechnology, food safety, and bioterrorism / Sari Edelstein ... [et al.].
    p.; cm.
  Includes bibliographical references and index.
  ISBN-13: 978-0-7637-5408-2 (pbk.)
  ISBN-10: 0-7637-5408-0 (pbk.)
    1. Food—United States—Safety measures. 2. Food contamination—United States. 3. Food—Biotechnology. 4. Foodborne diseases—United States. 5. Bioterrorism. I. Edelstein, Sari.
    [DNLM: 1. Food Industry—United States. 2. Safety Management—United States. 3. Bioterrorism—United States. 4. Food Contamination—United States. 5. Food Supply—economics—United States. 6. Food, Genetically Modified—United States. 7. Hunger—United States. WA 695 F68621 2009]
  RA601.F655 2009
  363.19′26—dc22
                                2008006663

6048

Printed in the United States of America
12 11 10 09 08 10 9 8 7 6 5 4 3 2 1

DEDICATION

To my husband, Marc, and my children, Staci, Jodi, and Sebastien.

Sari Edelstein

*To my husband Mike, my parents Peter and Charlotte Hackes,
and my brother Lee Miller.*

Bonnie Gerald

To my husband, Christian.

Tamara M. Crutchley Bushell

To my wife, Lisa, and my children, Diego, Faith, and Van.

Craig Gundersen

*Thanks to: Mike Brown, Katey Birtcher, Tracey Chapman,
and Dawn Browder.*

CONTENTS

Chapter 3:   **Safety Issues in the US Food System**   **41**

Bonnie L. Gerald, PhD, DTR

Chapter 4:   **Food Safety Regulations and Programs**   **57**

Bonnie L. Gerald, PhD, DTR

LIST OF TABLES

Table 1.1 Average Annual Hospitalizations and Deaths for Gastrointestinal Illness by Diagnostic Category, National Hospital Discharge Survey, 1992 to 1996

Table 1.2 Summary of Inventory for Federal Food Safety Research

Table 1.3 Percentage of Respondents Identifying Each Pathogen as among the Top Three Causes of Foodborne Illness and Estimated Percentage of Foodborne Illnesses in the United States Actually Caused by Those Pathogens

Table 2.1 Foods Implicated with Foodborne Illness

Table 2.2 Foodborne Illnesses

Table 2.3 Federal Agencies and Web Sites with Food Safety Responsibilities

Table 4.1 Federal Agency Food Safety Responsibilities

Table 5.1 Primary Packaging

Table 5.2 Genetically Modified Food Products: Benefits and Controversies

Table 6.1 Food Insecurity Questions in the Core Food Security Module

Table 6.2 Food Insecurity for American Indians and Non-American Indians

Table 6.3 Food Insecurity for American Indians and Non-American Indians, Households with Incomes Below 185% of the Poverty Line

Table 10.1 Foodborne Illness Outbreaks

LIST OF FIGURES

FOREWORD

Food seems simple. It is a necessary part of our lives every single day. When abundant, it is easy to take food for granted, but occasionally we are reminded of its importance and its costs. Questions related to food safety, security, and the implications of new technologies are complex ones. Students of food and nutrition, food science, and public health need to be skilled at considering complex questions. Is our food safe? This is a question that is on the minds of many consumers today. Food safety exists on several levels. Is our food free of pathogens? Is our food free of components that increase our risk for chronic disease? Does our food provide adequate amounts of essential nutrients and contain additional compounds that prevent disease and promote health?

Food dangers arise when food is scarce or when not everyone has safe or socially acceptable ways to access food. We need to strive for food security as families, communities, as a nation, and as a global society. There are different approaches to achieving global food security. Should every small village or community be self-reliant, producing food with limited inputs on a small scale? Or should we specialize and trade for foodstuffs, centralizing and industrializing food production and relying on inexpensive fuel to transport it? These strategies are both employed in the world today, as are many scenarios that fall somewhere in between.

The challenge for those in our food and healthcare systems is in determining where to strike a balance for maximum food safety and food security. When news reports tell of product recalls or foodborne illness outbreaks related to the industrial food system, many consumers start looking for food produced closer to home, by people they know. When midwinter limits the variety of local foods or when convenience is perceived as a necessity, consumers are in turn drawn toward the globally and industrially supplied supermarket.

It is easy to appreciate both the freshness and flavor of local food and the variety and convenience of industrial food. Students and professionals alike will be able to critically evaluate the advantages of each in view of their costs. The industrial food system, for example, has done much to ensure that we have an abundant and affordable supply of food, thus improving the quality of our lives. Which gains have been worth their costs (i.e., costs for the environment; costs for agricultural communities, culture, and traditions; and costs for our long-term public health)?

Understanding food issues entails understanding trade-offs on both personal and societal levels. When does having immediate food safety compromise our long-term health? Does selecting particular vegetable varieties that are durable for transportation compromise the nutrient density and flavor of the food? What intrinsic qualities of food are lost when they are mass produced? How has the mass production of a few crop varieties in monocultures threatened long-term food security, which is dependent on ecological diversity? How have our agricultural advances made the food system vulnerable to interruption by terrorists? When are sustainability, food safety, and food security at odds?

One of the roles for those charged with responsibilities for our food supply and nutritional status is helping individual clients as well as broader populations understand how to make good food choices. Having choices related to food is a blessing when we understand the power they hold. Our food choices determine, in part, how healthy we will be as individuals. They also can affect our communities and the surrounding landscape. Ultimately our food choices will shape the future food system, its safety, and security. What do we value about food? How do our choices enact those values? Food is not so simple after all. This text will be a tool to help educators train future food and nutrition professionals to critically consider complex questions about food safety, food security, food technology, and the food system as a whole. For those already at work in the field, this book will serve as a valuable reference concerning this most critical issue.

Alison Harmon, PhD, RD, LN
Health and Human Development
Montana State University

CHAPTER 1

IS AMERICA AT RISK?

Sari Edelstein, PhD, RD

Chapter Objectives

After reading the chapter and reflecting on the contents, you should be able to:

1. Identify the concern for food safety and the presence of food-borne illness in the United States.
2. Articulate an understanding of the term "biotechnology" as it relates to genetically modified food.
3. Determine that food insecurity is a growing problem in the United States.
4. Recognize that the threat of agroterrorism/bioterrorism exists in the United States

Key Terms

agroterrorism: Includes purposeful adulteration/poisoning of agricultural crops and the food supply to cause illness or death.
biotechnology: Includes a gene slicing technique that enables scientists to insert genes into foods for the purpose of dealing with the environmental stresses the world now poses.
bioterrorism: Includes purposeful adulteration/poisoning of food or food sources to cause illness or death.
food insecurity: Relates to the access to wholesome, healthy foods.
food safety: The pursuit of uncontaminated, unadulterated, clean, wholesome food that is fit for healthy consumption.
foodborne illness: A disease that is carried or transmitted to people by food. Pathogens in food can generate infection, intoxication, or intoxification.

genetically modified foods: Foods that have undergone gene slicing or gene replacement.

Introduction

This book, *Food and Nutrition at Risk in America: Food Insecurity,
Biotechnology, Food Safety, and Bioterrorism*, addresses the
strengths and weaknesses of four paramount issues in America's
struggle to provide *safe and adequate* food and nutrition for all
those living within its borders. As we leap into the second decade of
the 21st century, we find that providing US inhabitants with "safe
and adequate" food has become a daunting task. So daunting, in
fact, that we might be on the verge of "crisis management" in our
ability to protect our population from pathogens and chemicals that
invade our food supply as well as our capability to supply enough
affordable food to feed our people.

Food and Nutrition at Risk in America takes a four-pronged
approach to expose those areas in the food and nutrition domain
that have become increasingly vulnerable to the provision of safe
and adequate food and nutrition in the United States. These four
areas of concern are: food safety, biotechnology and genetically
modified foods, food insecurity, and agro/bioterrorism.

Food Safety

Food safety includes the pursuit of uncontaminated, unadulterated,
clean, wholesome food that is fit for healthy consumption. To feed
the population safe food, the food should not cause illness upon
ingestion or during the hours following ingestion. In short, safe
food should not cause a foodborne illness, which is a disease that is
carried or transmitted to people by food (FDA, 2006). Food safety
can be threatened by biological, chemical, or physical hazards. In
Section One of this book, biological foodborne pathogens, their etiology, and emerging pathogens in the US food system will be highlighted for the reader. Disease-causing pathogens in food can
generate infection, intoxication, or intoxification for unwitting consumers. These illnesses can cause morbidity and mortality at alarm-

ing rates. Table 1.1 indicates illness rates from biological foodborne illness in the United States.

Table 1.2 gives an account of the current dollars spent by the United States in three of its major governmental offices—US Department of Agriculture (USDA), US Department of Health and Human Services (HHS), and Environmental Protection Agency (EPA)—on food safety programs. Table 1.3 lists the percentage of respondents who identified various pathogens as the top three causes of foodborne illnesses and the estimated percentage of US foodborne illnesses that were actually caused by those pathogens.

Figure 1.1 depicts the surveillance rates from 1996 to 2004 of five major foodborne illnesses, and Figure 1.2 indicates the five types of *Salmonella* infection rates from those years.

Chemical hazards in food are linked to paint, lubricants, cleaning agents, and pesticides while physical hazards include broken glass, metal shavings, and plastic ties. These hazards should not be minimized in their importance of control in the food supply. *Food and Nutrition at Risk in America* will focus on biological hazards as the major source of foodborne illness in the United States.

Table 1.1 Average Annual Hospitalizations and Deaths for Gastrointestinal Illness by Diagnostic Category, National Hospital Discharge Survey, 1992 to 1996

	First diagnosis		All diagnoses	
Cause of enteritis[a]	Hospitalizations	Deaths	Hospitalizations	Deaths
Bacterial (001–005, 008–008.5)	27,987	148[b]	54,953	1,139
Viral (008.6–008.8)	82,149	0[b]	132,332	194[b]
Parasitic (006–007)	2,806	8?[b]	5,799	127[b]
Unknown etiology (009, 558.9)	186,537	868[b]	423,293	5,148
Total	299,479	1,098	616,377	6,608

[a]ICD-9-CM code.
[b]Estimate unreliable due to small sample size.

Source: Mead, P.S., Slutsker, L., Dietz, V., McCaig, L.F., Bresee, J.S., Shapiro C., et al. (1999). Food-related illness and death in the United States. *Emerging Infectious Diseases Newsletter*, Vol. 5, No. 5. Retrieved October 12, 2007, from http://www.cdc.gov/ncidod/eid/vol5no5/mead.htm.

Table 1.2 Summary of Inventory for Federal Food Safety Research

	Fiscal Year 2000, Dollars in 1,000s (Estimated)							
	HHS		USDA		EPA		Total[a]	
Research focus	Projects	Dollars	Projects	Dollars	Projects	Dollars	Projects	Dollars
Detection of foodborne hazards	54	23,365		19,846		900		
Control of foodborne hazards	8	3,700		51,325		0		
Pathogenicity of foodborne microbes	16	7,400		0		0		
Antimicrobial/antibiotic resistance/ susceptibility of foodborne microbes	8	3,900		8,115		0		
Epidemiology of food-associated organisms/illness	5	200		7,000		2,000		
Risk assessment: methods/data	7	3,177		10,011		600		
Food handling, distribution, and storage	0	0		12,791		0		
Economic analysis	0	0		3,230		0		
Total		123,099[a]		112,318		3,500[b]		238,917

[a]This number includes $81,357 million for National Institutes of Health (NIH), whose research dollars are not allocated until after grant awards are actually made; splits reflect only Centers for Disease Control and Prevention (CDC) and Food and Drug Administration (FDA) dollars, and no totals are given by category.
[b]Funding levels for the EPA competitive grants program in fiscal year 2000 that is specifically targeted to drinking water pathogen research have not been determined at this time.

Source: USDA Food Safety Research Information Office. (2005). Retrieved September 20, 2007, from http://fsrio.nal.usda.gov/.

Table 1.3   Percentage of Respondents Identifying Each Pathogen as among the Top Three Causes of Foodborne Illness and Estimated Percentage of Foodborne Illnesses in the United States Actually Caused by Those Pathogens

Pathogen	Percentage of respondents listing it among top three causes	Estimated percentage of foodborne illness in United States caused by pathogen
Salmonella	90	9.7
Escherichia coli	56	1.3
Staphylococcus	36	1.3
Shigella	32	0.6
Campylobacter	18	14.2
Listeria	16	<0.1
Hepatitis A virus	8	<0.1
Clostridium perfringens	8	1.8
Norwalk-like virus	5	66.7
Viruses[a]	4	67.2
Giardia lamblia	3	1.4
Streptococcus	2	0.4

[a]This represents respondents who wrote in "viruses" only; it does not include those who specified Norwalk-like virus.

Source: Jones, T.F., & Gerber, D.E. (2001). Perceived etiology of foodborne illness among public health personnel. *Emerging Infectious Diseases Newsletter*, Vol. 7, No. 5. Retrieved October 12, 2007, from http://www.cdc.gov/ncidod/eid/vol7no5/jones.htm.

Biotechnology and Genetically Modified Foods

Biotechnology includes a gene slicing technique that enables scientists to insert genes into foods for the purpose of dealing with the environmental stresses the world now poses (Bren, 2003). Figure 1.3 illustrates gene slicing. The result is a *genetically modified food* that should be better able to withstand environmental stresses and provide people with higher quality and quantity of food. More than 50 genetically modified food products have been evaluated by the FDA and were found to be as safe as conventional foods, including canola oil, corn, cottonseed oil, papaya, potatoes, soybeans, squash, sugar beets, sweet corn, and tomatoes. Figure 1.4 depicts the percentage of

FIGURE 1.1   Relative Rates Compared with 1996 to 1998 Baseline Period of Laboratory-Diagnosed Cases of Infection with *Campylobacter, Escherichia coli* O157, *Listeria, Salmonella,* and *Vibrio,* by Year—Foodborne Diseases Active Surveillance Network, United States, 1996 to 2004

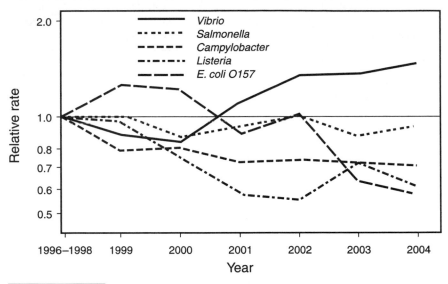

Source: CDC. (2005). Preliminary FoodNet data on the incidence of infection with pathogens transmitted commonly through food—10 sites, United States, 2004. (MMWR, Vol. 54, No. 14, pp. 352–356.) Retrieved September 20, 2007, from http://www.cdc.gov/mmwr/preview/mmwrhtml/mm5414a2.htm#tab.

genetically modified soybeans, corn, and cotton that now exist in our crop supply.

Food Insecurity

Food insecurity encompasses many categories of persons within the United States, which include those who are food insecure without hunger and food insecure with hunger. Chapter 6 gives insight to the differences between these terms and how they are determined in the United States. As of 2002, the USDA reports that some 11% of US households experienced food insecurity (Nord, Andrews, & Carlson, 2002). This is a rise from past years and represents a threat to US health. Figure 1.5 depicts the percentage of food insecurity by type in the United States.

FIGURE 1.2 Relative Rates Compared with 1996 to 1998 Baseline Period of Laboratory-Diagnosed Cases of Infection with the Five Most Commonly Isolated *Salmonella* Serotypes, by Year—Foodborne Diseases Active Surveillance Network, United States, 1996 to 2004

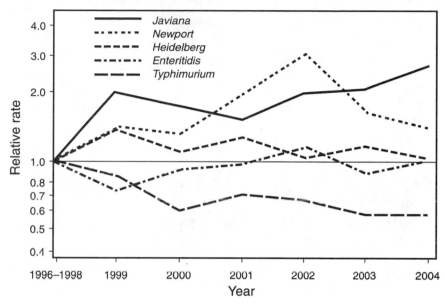

Source: CDC. (2005). Preliminary FoodNet data on the incidence of infection with pathogens transmitted commonly through food—10 Sites, United States, 2004. (MMWR, Vol. 54, No. 14, pp. 352 356.) Retrieved September 20, 2007, from http://www.cdc.gov/mmwr/preview/mmwrhtml/mm5414a2.htm#tab.

Food and Nutrition at Risk in America will delineate some solutions for food insecurity through federal, state, and community assistance programs. While these programs are vital to the health of the US people, cost and cause must be analyzed further.

Agro/Bioterrorism

Agro/bioterrorism includes purposeful adulteration/poisoning of food to cause illness or death. Although acts of aggression against the US food supply are not new, 9/11 made the potential a possible reality both within the United States and from outside perpetrators. The United States established the Bioterrorism Act of 2002 to delineate where threats would occur and our preparedness (USDA, 2002).

FIGURE 1.3   Traditional Plant Breeding and Modern Plant Breeding
(Genetic Engineering)

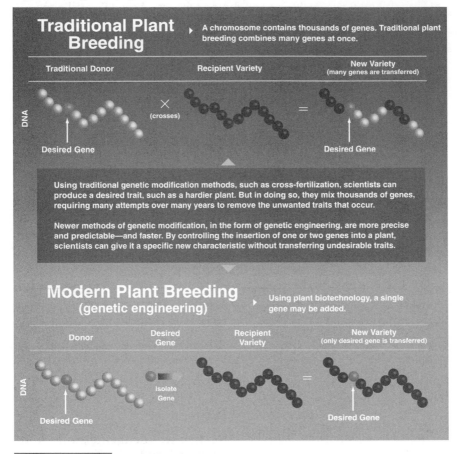

Source: Bren, L. (2003). Genetic engineering: The future of foods? *FDA Consumer Magazine,*
November–December. Retrieved October 12, 2007, from http://www.fda.gov/fdac/features/
2003/plantDNA.html.

The act includes the following five titles and can be found in complete form at http://www.fda.gov/oc/bioterrorism/PL107-188.html:

  Title I—National Preparedness for Bioterrorism and Other Public
      Health Emergencies
  Title II—Enhancing Controls on Dangerous Biological Agents
      and Toxins
  Title III—Protecting Safety and Security of Food and Drug
      Supply

FIGURE 1.4   Top Three Genetically Engineered Crops in the United States (2003)

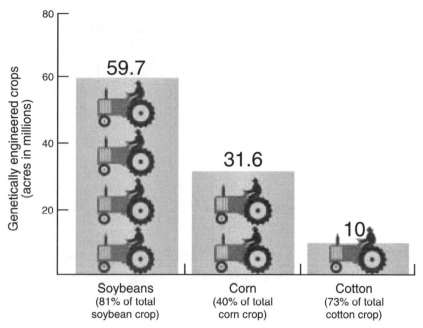

Source: National Agricultural Statistics Service/USDA

Source: Bren, L. (2003). Genetic engineering: The future of foods? *FDA Consumer Magazine,* November–December. Retrieved October 12, 2007, from http://www.fda.gov/fdac/features/2003/603_food.html.

Title IV—Drinking Water Security and Safety
Title V—Additional Provisions

In addition to the policy making of the USDA, the FDA (n.d.) is working to prevent acts of bioterrorism through:

- working with industry to reduce threats and contain outbreaks of foodborne illness
- increasing risk-based surveillance of domestic and imported food
- developing *PrepNet* food safety network
- implementing the Bioterrorism Act of 2002
- increasing the ability to quickly identify outbreaks of foodborne illness
- increasing participation in the first Internet-based food safety system

FIGURE 1.5   US Households by Security Status, 2002

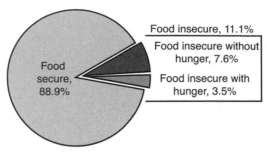

Source: Calculated by ERS using data from the December 2002
Current Population Survey Food Security Supplement.

Source: Nord, M., Andrews, M., & Carlson, S. (2002). *Household food security in the United States, 2002.* Retrieved October 12, 2007, from www.ers.usda.gov/Publications/FANRR35/.

Food and Nutrition at Risk in America will clarify the risk for the reader as well as the state of preparedness of the United States.

Issues to Debate

1. How educated do you think the public is about these topics at the present time?
2. Why do you think that the public is or is not informed about these topics?
3. How important is each of these topics?
4. Is the US government doing enough to solve the food and nutrition problems of the country?
5. Rate the importance of each topic against one another and place them in order of importance. Explain your results.

Web Sites

US FDA/Center for Food Safety and Applied Nutrition
www.cfsan.fda.gov/

FDA's food biotechnology Web site
www.cfsan.fda.gov/~lrd/biotechm.html

List of bioengineered foods that have completed FDA consultation
www.cfsan.fda.gov

USDA's report on household food security
www.ers.usda.gov/Publications/FANRR35/

Bioterrorism and food safety
www.foodsafety.gov/~fsg/bioterr.html

Bioterrorism Act of 2002
http://www.fda.gov/oc/bioterrorism/PL107-188.html

FDA's role in bioterrorism
http://www.fda.gov/oc/bioterrorism/role.html

US Department of Agriculture Food Safety and Inspection Service
http://www.fsis.usda.gov/PDF/Food_Defense_Plan.pdf

References

Bren, L. (2003). Genetic engineering: The future of foods? *FDA Consumer Magazine*, November–December. Retrieved October 12, 2007, from http://www.fda.gov/fdac/features/2003/603_food.html

Food and Drug Administration. (n.d.). *FDA's counterterrorism role*. Retrieved October 12, 2007, from http://www.fda.gov/oc/bioterrorism/role.html

Food and Drug Administration, Center for Food Safety and Applied Nutrition. (2006, April 25). *Foodborne pathogenic microorganisms and natural toxins handbook (Bad bug book)*. Retrieved September 20, 2007, from http://vm.cfsan.fda.gov/~mow/intro.html

Nord, M., Andrews, M., & Carlson, S. (2002). *Household food security in the United States, 2002*. Retrieved October 12, 2007, from www.ers.usda.gov/Publications/FANRR35/

USDA. (2002). *Bioterrorism act of 2002*. Retrieved October 12, 2007, from http://www.fda.gov/oc/bioterrorism/PL107-188.html

SECTION ONE

FOOD SAFETY AND BIOTECHNOLOGY

CHAPTER 2

FOODBORNE ILLNESS-CAUSING PATHOGENS

Bonnie L. Gerald, PhD, DTR

Chapter Objectives

After reading the chapter and reflecting on the contents, you should be able to:

1. Define the three categories of illness-causing pathogens.
2. Identify potential pathogens for different types of food and beverages.
3. Articulate typical symptoms of foodborne illness.
4. Delineate proactive measures to decrease risk of foodborne illness.
5. Identify pathogens that can be future sources of foodborne illness outbreaks.

Key Terms

foodborne illness: Illness caused by a food hosting an undesired physical, chemical, or bacterial agent.

foodborne illness infection: Occurs when pathogens grow in the intestines of the person who consumes the pathogen-contaminated food.

foodborne illness intoxication: Caused by eating toxins produced by the pathogen already in the food.

foodborne illness intoxification: Occurs when pathogens are ingested and produce toxins in the intestines.

pathogen: Virus, bacteria, parasite, or other agent that causes disease.

spp.: Species.

Introduction

Foodborne illness has caused both significant health and financial burdens to the US population. The Centers for Disease Control and Prevention (CDC) estimates there are 76 million reported cases of foodborne illness annually, with a more than $400 billion impact (Frenzen, Drake, & Angulo, 2005). Each case of foodborne illness can result in lost wages and increased medical costs, and it can be a source of misery for the affected individual. The symptoms can last for several hours to several years, depending on the pathogen and source of contact. Foodborne pathogens can be present at each stage in the food system, from the farm to the consumer's table. Therefore, it is important to have the ability to recognize potential sources of contamination, identify the symptoms of foodborne illness, and be proactive in implementing food safety practices.

What is a foodborne illness? According to the Center for Food Safety and Applied Nutrition (CFSAN), it is a disease that is carried or transmitted to people by food (Food and Drug Administration, Center for Food Safety and Applied Nutrition [FDA], 2006). A case of foodborne illness refers to one person becoming ill; a foodborne illness outbreak occurs when two or more people become ill after eating the same food (FDA, 2006). Foods can become unsafe due to biological, chemical, or physical hazards. Chemicals such as paint, lubricants, cleaning agents, and pesticides can make people sick. Physical hazards such as broken glass, metal shavings, and plastic ties can cause injury when ingested. Food producers/processors who implement standard operating procedures (SOPs), such as preventive maintenance, sanitation, and inspection programs, will minimize the risk from chemical and physical hazards. Biological hazards, which include bacteria, viruses, and parasites, are the major source of foodborne illness in the United States. This chapter will focus on identification of the major foodborne pathogens and their etiology, and it will describe several emerging pathogens in the US food system.

Disease-causing pathogens can generate infection, intoxication, or intoxification. An infection occurs when pathogens grow in the intestines of the person who consumes the pathogen-contaminated food. Intoxication is caused by eating toxins produced by the pathogen. An intoxification illness occurs when pathogens are ingested and produce toxins in the intestines (Brown, 2005). Molds, yeasts, and fungi cause food spoilage. Consuming spoiled food can cause illness; however, this is unlikely to occur. Spoiled food differs from pathogen-contaminated food in that the presence of spoilage microorganisms produce visual and olfactory evidence that they are spoiled.

Although there is a wide range of foodborne illness-causing pathogens, they all have similar needs to support their growth. An effective technique to remember these conditions is the acronym FAT TOM. Pathogens require food (F), usually proteins and carbohydrates. The pH should be in the neutral range, typically 4.6 to 7.5. Highly acidic or alkaline (A) foods do not support microbial growth. The temperature range of 41°F to 135°F is where most pathogens live and multiply, sometimes at a geometric rate. This temperature range is known as the temperature danger zone (T). Time (T) is needed for pathogens to reproduce to hazardous levels. Some microorganisms can double their population in 20 minutes. Oxygen (O) is a determining factor of the type of pathogen growth. Some microorganisms require oxygen (aerobic); some microorganisms cannot reproduce in the presence of oxygen (anaerobic); others can grow with or without oxygen (facultative). Most of the foodborne illness-causing pathogens are facultative (FDA, 2006). Pathogens also require water for growth. In general, high moisture (M) foods support foodborne illness-causing pathogens. The amount of water in food is measured by its water activity (aw), or the proportion of water freely available in a food compared to distilled water. On a scale of 0 (no water) to 1.0 (distilled water), foods with water activity of 0.85 or above are likely to become hazardous.

Assuming the conditions for pathogen growth are present, which situations are most likely to create unsafe food? Most incidents of pathogen-caused foodborne illness can be attributed to cross contamination, poor personal hygiene, and time–temperature abuse. Cross contamination occurs when a pathogen-contaminated surface contacts an uncontaminated surface, thus transferring the pathogens. Examples of cross contamination are using the same cutting board to slice vegetables after cutting up a chicken or making potato salad in the same container in which raw ground

Learning Point: Foods can become unsafe due to biological, chemical, or physical hazards.

beef was stored. Poor personal hygiene can range from improper hand washing, preparing food with an open wound, or coming to work with diarrhea. The probability of foodborne illness-causing pathogens occurring on food is likely when the above conditions have been met.

Types of Pathogens: Bacteria

Bacteria are the most prevalent form of foodborne illness-causing pathogens. They are living, one-celled microorganisms that can be carried by food, humans, water, soil, animals, and insects. Approximately 4% of all bacteria are pathogenic, while the remaining 96% are harmless (FDA, 2006). Food infections and food intoxications (i.e., "food poisoning") are the most common forms of bacterial foodborne illness, with infections accounting for 80% of foodborne illness. The most common bacterial infections result from *Listeria monocytogenes*, *Salmonella* spp., *Shigella* spp., *Streptococcus pyogenes*, and *Yersinia enterocolitica*. Bacterial intoxications are caused by *Clostridium botulinum*, *Clostridium perfringens*, *Bacillus cereus*, and *Staphylococcus aureus*. Bacterial intoxifications, the foodborne illness caused by bacteria colonizing the intestines and then producing toxins, are generated by *Escherichia coli*, *Campylobacter jejuni*, *Vibrio parahaemolyticus*, and *Vibrio vulnificus*.

Bacterial Infection: *Listeria monocytogenes*

Listeria monocytogenes is a facultative bacterium that is capable of growing in wide temperature (39°F to 113°F) and pH (4.8 to 9.0) ranges. *Listeria* bacteria can be found in soil, water, and intestinal tracts of humans and animals. It has been linked to foodborne illness from frozen dairy desserts, milk, Mexican-style soft cheese, luncheon meats, and cabbage. The incubation period is typically 3 weeks. Listeriosis presents as nausea, vomiting, persistent fever, chills, and backache. Severe cases can result in encephalitis, meningitis, septicemia, and cervical infections. Listeriosis can last for indefinite periods, depending on treatment (FDA, 2006). Fatality rates can range from 20% to 35% of those infected. FoodNet, CDC's Foodborne Diseases Active Surveillance Network, estimates that incidents of listeriosis declined 34% in 2006 from the 1996 to 1998

> **Learning Point:** Pregnant women, fetuses, and infants are the most vulnerable to listeriosis.

baseline period (Centers for Disease Control [CDC], 2007a). Control measures include cooking foods to the appropriate temperature, avoiding cross contamination, and using only pasteurized dairy products.

Bacterial Infection: *Salmonella* spp.

Salmonellosis is caused by a wide variety of *Salmonella* serotypes. *Salmonella typhimurium* is the most common serotype. It is a non-spore-forming, facultative bacteria capable of surviving pH below 4.5. *Salmonella* are present in cattle, poultry, eggs, raw milk, water, and soil. The incubation period ranges from 6–48 hours. Salmonellosis is more common in summer than winter. Symptoms include abdominal cramps, nausea, fever, and diarrhea that lasts for 1–2 days. Children are the most susceptible to the disease. Approximately 40,000 cases of salmonellosis are reported in the United States annually (CDC, 2005a). FoodNet data indicate a decline in *Salmonella typhimurium* in 2006 from the baseline period, but no significant changes in the incidence of other *Salmonella* serotypes (CDC, 2007a). *Salmonella* can be controlled by cooking all red meat, poultry, and eggs thoroughly; using pasteurized milk and egg products; using water from approved sources; and thoroughly washing all produce. However, washing might not remove all *Salmonella* bacteria (FDA, 2007a; FDA, 2007b).

> **Learning Point:** Recent outbreaks of salmonellosis from spinach, lettuce, and tomatoes indicate the need for improved sanitation in produce harvesting and packing operations (CDC, 2005a; FDA, 2007a; FDA, 2007b).

Bacterial Infection: *Shigella* spp.

Shigella is a non-spore-forming facultative bacteria that can produce toxins in some serotypes. About 18,000 cases of shigellosis are reported annually; however, the CDC estimates the actual number of

> **Learning Point:** *Shigella* is most prevalent in winter, causing the majority of infections among 2- to 4-year-old children.

cases might be 20 times higher (CDC, 2005b). Shigellosis is highly contagious and can spread through entire communities. Symptoms typically appear in 1–3 days and can last for up to 7 days. Shigellosis is characterized by diarrhea, fever, nausea, cramps, and sometimes vomiting. Raw foods are typical sources of contamination; however, the *Shigella* bacteria are spread to foods by human feces or fecal-contaminated water. Good personal hygiene, especially proper hand washing, is an effective method of control. Community water and sewage treatment is also an effective control measure. The CDC estimates that shigellosis declined 50% in 2006 compared to the baseline period 1996 to 1998 (CDC, 2007a).

Bacterial Infection: *Streptococcus pyogenes*

Streptococcus bacteria present a moderate risk to human health with the potential for widespread infection in the population. The incubation period is 1–3 days, presenting as sore throat, erysipelas, and scarlet fever. Persons with sore throats or other strep infections also

> **Learning Point:** Sources of the bacteria *Streptococcus* are raw milk and eggs.

can spread the disease (FDA, 2006; Brown, 2005). The bacteria can be controlled by good sanitation practices and using only pasteurized milk products.

Bacterial Infection: *Yersinia enterocolitica*

Yersinia enterocolitica is a non-spore-forming facultative bacteria that is capable of surviving in low temperatures and pH below 4.5. The yersiniosis incubation period is 3–7 days, with a duration of 2–3 weeks. However, it can become chronic in some individuals. Symptoms of yersiniosis can mimic appendicitis and also can include headache, sore throat, diarrhea, and vomiting. Cooking meat to the appropriate temperature and using chlorine-treated water are meth-

> **Learning Point:** Raw or undercooked red meat, oysters, water, and tofu are common sources of *Yersinia* infections.

ods to control yersiniosis (National Restaurant Education Foundation, 2005; FDA, 2006). The incidence of *Yersinia* infections has declined 50% since the 1996 to 1998 baseline period (CDC, 2007a).

Bacterial Intoxication: *Clostridium botulinum*

Clostridium botulinum is a rod-shaped, spore-forming anaerobic bacteria. The spores are widespread due to water and dust and can be present on most foods. Canned, low-acid foods, garlic in oil products, cooked meats, and fish are common sources. Home canned products such as green beans are at risk for carrying the pathogen. Any food that has been undercooked or time–temperature abused is capable of supporting *Clostridium botulinum* growth. Botulism affects the nervous system, presenting as fatigue, double vision, slurred speech, and respiratory failure. Severe cases can cause death. Although the reported incidence is low (110 cases per year), botulism is considered to be a serious medical condition. Because of the very small amount of bacteria needed to generate the disease, botulism is one of the deadliest foodborne illnesses (FDA, 2006). *Clostridium botulinum* bacteria can be controlled by appropriate heating and cooling of foods (CDC, 2005c).

> **Learning Point:** Infants are susceptible to botulism from raw honey.

Bacterial Intoxication: *Clostridium perfringens*

Clostridium perfringens is a spore-forming, anaerobic bacteria found in soil and raw foods. Consumption of improperly cooked or cooled meats, poultry, gravies, or foods contaminated by *Clostridium*-containing dust (such as on the tops of cans) can lead to an intoxication. The incubation period is 8–24 hours, and the disease typically lasts for 12–24 hours. Symptoms include diarrhea, nausea, abdominal pain, and dehydration. *Clostridium perfringens* intoxications are considered to be a moderate hazard that is self-limiting (FDA, 2006; National Restaurant Association Educational Foundation, 2005). Using appropriate time and temperature control of cooked, cooled, or reheated foods will decrease the risk of *Clostridium perfringens* intoxication.

Bacterial Intoxication: *Bacillus cereus*

Bacillus cereus is a spore-forming, facultative bacteria. There are two forms of the disease: emetic and diarrheal. Both forms originate from soil or dust. The emetic form has a rapid onset, from 30 minutes to 6 hours, and presents as nausea, vomiting, and occasional diarrhea for 5–24 hours. The diarrheal form has a latency period of 6–15 hours and lasts from 12–24 hours. Diarrheal symptoms include diarrhea, cramps, and occasional vomiting. Time and temperature abused cooked rice and pasta favor the growth of emetic *Bacillus cereus* bacteria. Disease incidence can be controlled by proper time and temperature control of cooked, cooled, and reheated foods. The CDC considers *Bacillus cereus* intoxication to be a mild illness (Mead et al., 1999).

> **Learning Point:** Cooked meats, vegetables, fish, and milk can harbor diarrheal *Bacillus cereus* bacteria (FDA, 2006).

Bacterial Intoxication: *Staphylococcus aureus*

Staphylococcus aureus is a non-spore-forming, facultative bacteria that can survive pH of 2.6 and is resistant to drying and freezing. Staphylococcal bacteria are commonly found on the human skin and nasal passages. The bacteria also are responsible for most minor skin infections in the United States and can cause serious bloodstream and wound infections. Intoxication onset is rapid, from 30 minutes to 8 hours after ingesting the toxin. Staphylococcal food poisoning typically lasts from 6–48 hours and is characterized by nausea, vomiting, cramps, and diarrhea (National Restaurant Association Educational Foundation, 2005; FDA, 2006). Practicing good personal hygiene and appropriate heating and cooling of foods will decrease the risk of staphylococcal food poisoning. The number of outbreak-associated cases of staphylococcal food poisoning has declined since the 1970s (Mead et al., 1999).

> **Learning Point:** Staphylococcal bacteria are transmitted to food by persons with skin infections or by touching the face, hair, and nasal passages while preparing food.

Bacterial Intoxification: *Escherichia coli*

Escherichia coli is a non-spore-forming facultative bacteria that is capable of growing under refrigeration temperatures and surviving in a pH 4.0 environment. *E. coli* bacteria are commonly found in the intestinal tracts of humans and animals. Manure or untreated sewage can contaminate water. *E. coli* is most frequently associated with undercooked ground beef, but it also has been linked to unpasteurized milk, unpasteurized juice, cider, raw sprouts, spinach, and lettuce. Different strains cause different illnesses, such as infant diarrhea, traveler's diarrhea, and bloody diarrhea. Children are particularly at risk for *E. coli* intoxifications. Another serious illness resulting from *E. coli* is Hemolytic Uremic Syndrome (HUS). HUS is the leading cause of renal failure in children (FDA, 2006). *E. coli* 0157:H7 is a virulent strain first detected in the 1980s. In 1993, the 0157:H7 strain was linked to several deaths from undercooked ground beef, the first confirmed mortality from the bacterial strain.

The CDC estimates that 73,000 cases of infection and 61 deaths occur annually (CDC, 2006a). The economic burden of *E. coli* 0157:H7 medical costs to lost productivity is $405 million annually (Frenzen, Drake, & Angulo, 2005). Depending on the strain, the incubation period is 10–72 hours with a duration of 2–9 days. If HUS develops, treatment in an intensive care unit is necessary. Some people with HUS can have lifelong complications such as blindness, paralysis, and kidney failure (CDC, 2006a). In 2002 a test for detecting *E. coli* 0157:H7 in ground beef was developed. However, the incidence of *E. coli* 0157:H7 infections did not decrease significantly in 2006 compared to the CDC's baseline reporting period (CDC, 2007a).

> **Learning Point:** A serious illness resulting from *E. coli* is Hemolytic Uremic Syndrome (HUS).

Bacterial Infection: *Campylobacter jejuni*

Campylobacter jejuni is a non-spore-forming bacteria. Campylobacteriosis accounts for more foodborne illness than salmonellosis (14.2% versus 9.7%, respectively) (Mead et al., 1999). Common sources of the bacteria are unpasteurized milk, improperly treated surface water, undercooked poultry, domestic animals, and wild animals. The onset of symptoms in about 2–5 days includes diarrhea, abdominal pain, fever, nausea, and vomiting; the duration is approximately 2–10 days (FDA, 2006). The incidence of campylobacteriosis has declined 30% from the baseline period (CDC, 2007a). The number of people infected annually in the United States is 1.7–2.45 million (Samuel et al., 2004).

Learning Point: The purchase of irradiated chicken, thoroughly cooking chicken, and using pasteurized milk are control measures for the transmission of campylobacteriosis.

Bacterial Intoxification: *Vibrio vulnificus, Vibrio parahaemolyticus*

Vibrio spp. is a non-spore-forming bacteria in the same family that causes cholera. The majority of reported foodborne illness occurs in the summer months. The most common source of *Vibrio* bacteria is oysters and other shellfish, especially from the Gulf of Mexico. *V. vulnificus* and *V. parahaemolyticus* are halophilic, requiring salt for survival. *V. parahaemolyticus* is the source of the majority of *Vibrio* intoxifications (CDC, 2005d; CDC, 2005e). The bacteria also can enter the body through skin wounds during harvesting and cleaning shellfish. The incubation period ranges from 4–38 hours with a duration of 1 day to several weeks. The illness presents as fever, chills, headache, cramps, diarrhea, and sometimes vomiting. Severe cases in immunocompromised persons can result in septicemia, decreased blood pressure, and death. Freezing shellfish does not destroy the bacteria. Approximately 5% to 10% of raw shellfish are contaminated (FDA, 2006). The incidence of *Vibrio* intoxifications increased 78% in 2006 compared to the 1996 to 1998 baseline data (CDC, 2007a).

Learning Point: Avoiding raw or undercooked seafood and purchasing seafood from reputable purveyors are control methods for *Vibrio* spp.

Types of Pathogens: Viruses

Viruses require a living host for survival. The smallest microbial contaminant, the virus's genetic material, has a protein layer as protection (National Restaurant Association Educational Foundation, 2005). All foodborne illness-causing viruses are transmitted by the fecal–oral route. The transmission can be from person to person or by fecal contaminated food, clothing, water, and flies (Brown, 2005). Viruses are not reproduced in food. Although foodborne viral illness is reported less often than bacterial foodborne illness, the severity can be greater and last longer. The major foodborne illness-causing viruses are hepatitis A, *Norovirus*, and *Rotavirus*. The resulting illness is called viral gastroenteritis, an inflammation of the stomach and large and small intestines. It is sometimes called "stomach flu"; however, it is not caused by influenza viruses (CDC, 2006b).

Viral Gastroenteritis: *Norovirus*

Norovirus refers to a group of nonenveloped, single-strand RNA viruses. The term "*Norovirus*" has replaced the previous designation of "Norwalk-like" viruses. This group of viruses belongs to the *Calicivirus* family. *Sapovirus* is another group belonging to the *Calicivirus* family that causes gastroenteritis. The fecal–oral route is the main source of transmission of foodborne illness. *Norovirus* outbreaks have been associated with salads, sandwiches, raspberries, bakery items, and oysters. Contaminated water also can harbor *Noroviruses*. The incubation period ranges from 10–50 hours presenting as acute-onset vomiting; watery, nonbloody diarrhea; abdominal cramps; and nausea. Recovery occurs in 1–3 days (CDC, 2006b). The virus is resistant to freezing, high temperatures, and 10 ppm chlorine-treated water. However, the CDC recommends appropriate time–temperature control, frequent hand washing, and using sick leave as effective control methods. The CDC estimates that 23 million cases, or 50%, of gastroenteritis are caused by *Noroviruses* (CDC, 2005f).

> **Learning Point:** *Norovirus* outbreaks have been associated with salads, sandwiches, raspberries, bakery items, oysters, and contaminated water.

Viral Gastroenteritis: *Rotavirus*

Rotavirus is a wheellike structure composed of nonenveloped, double-shelled RNA. The virus is the most common cause of severe diarrhea among children, resulting in hospitalization of 55,000 children annually. *Rotavirus* has a winter seasonal pattern. The fecal–oral route is the main mode of transmission (CDC, 2007b). *Rotavirus* outbreaks are associated with water, ice, salads, and sandwiches. The virus will incubate for 1–3 days and last for 3–10 days. Temporary immunity from *Rotavirus* can occur for several months. Symptoms include nausea, vomiting, mild fever, and abdominal pain. Control measures are similar to *Noroviruses*: good personal hygiene, appropriate time–temperature control, and using water from approved sources. There is a vaccine to protect infants and young children from severe diarrhea resulting from *Rotavirus* infections (CDC, 2006b).

Viral Infections: Hepatitis A Virus (HAV)

Hepatitis A is the viral infection resulting from hepatitis A virus (HAV). It is a picornavirus with primates as the only host. The CDC estimates that 263,000 cases of hepatitis A occurred annually during the 1980 to 2001 period, declining slightly after 1999 (Fiore, 2004). Infection occurs through the fecal–oral route. Symptoms of fever, anorexia, nausea, vomiting, diarrhea, and myalgia appear after an incubation period of 10–50 days. The peak infectivity period occurs before jaundice, dark colored urine, or light colored stools present. Hepatitis A lasts for 1–2 weeks in the majority of cases. However, persons with chronic liver disease and the elderly can have extended illness and potential relapses, resulting in death in 1.8% of cases.

Food can be contaminated at any stage in the food system, making positive identification of an HAV source difficult. Foods that are not heated before service can harbor the virus, such as vegetables, sandwiches, and seafood. Water and ice and transmit the virus to humans. Practicing good personal hygiene, preventing cross contamination, and using appropriate sanitation procedures will help prevent the spread of HAV (National Restaurant Association Educational Foundation, 2005). A postexposure vaccine is effective if given within 2 weeks of exposure to HAV. Most individuals become immune to HAV after exposure to the virus. The CDC estimates that approximately 30% of the US population has HAV antigens (Fiore, 2004).

> **Learning Point:** Practicing good personal hygiene, preventing cross contamination, and using appropriate sanitation procedures will help prevent the spread of viruses.

Types of Pathogens: Parasites

Like viruses, parasites need a living host to survive. Parasites are microscopic organisms that are slightly larger than bacteria. Parasites can use several types of hosts, such as plants and animals, to complete their life cycle. Most cases of parasite-caused foodborne illness are passed to humans by animals. Both food and water can be contaminated with parasites. Two types of foodborne illness causing parasites are roundworms and protozoa (FDA, 2006; Brown, 2005). Parasitic foodborne illness accounts for approximately 3% of total reported foodborne illness; however, parasites are responsible for 21% of all foodborne illness-related deaths (Mead et al., 1999).

Parasitic Roundworms: *Trichinella spiralis*

The incidence of trichinellosis (also called trichinosis) in the United States has declined; 12 cases per year were reported in the period 1997 to 2001, the most recent available statistics (CDC, 2005g). The *Trichinella* worms are ingested from raw or undercooked meat. Stomach acid dissolves the worm's outer capsule, allowing the worms to colonize the small intestine. The eggs of the mature worms travel through the host's arteries and become lodged in muscle tissue. A cyst then encloses the worm within the muscle, thus infecting the host.

Symptoms occurring 1–2 days after infection include nausea, fever, diarrhea, abdominal pain, and swelling around the eyes. Approximately 2–8 weeks after consuming the infected meat, the victim might experience fatigue, sweating, chills, muscle soreness, and hemorrhaging (FDA, 2006). Trichinellosis is not contagious. Prescription drugs can successfully treat trichinellosis after diagnosis.

The risk of infection can be decreased by thoroughly cooking meat to the temperature recommended by the Food Code (FDA, 2005).

Learning Point: Pork and wild game meats are the most common sources of trichinellosis; however, all meat can be infected. Cooking utensils and sausage-making equipment should be thoroughly cleaned and sanitized (FDA, 2005).

Parasitic Roundworms: *Anisakis simplex* and *Pseudoterranova decipiens*

A. simplex and *P. decipiens* are parasites of marine fish. Persons consuming raw or undercooked fish are susceptible to infection. The worms are extremely small and can be missed by cooks who prepare sushi or sashimi dishes. There is currently no reliable method of detecting worms in fish. A tingling feeling might be present as the infected fish is swallowed. Symptoms can appear in 1 hour to 2 weeks after consumption and include nausea, vomiting, abdominal pain, and cramping. After several weeks the worm dies or can be vomited up. In severe cases the worm can penetrate the stomach or intestinal wall. Physicians can detect the worm in the stomach by using a fiber optic device and then using a forceps device to remove the worm (FDA, 2006). The parasites can be destroyed by freezing the fish at 4°F or colder for at least 7 days. Seafood should be purchased only from certified sources. Cooking fish and shellfish to the appropriate Food Code temperature also will control the parasites (FDA, 2005). Acidic marinades will not kill *Anisakis simplex*.

Learning Point: Persons who consume raw or undercooked fish are susceptible to infection by *A. simplex* and *P. decipiens*.

Parasitic Protozoa: *Giardia lamblia*

Protozoa are one-celled animals that infect humans through drinking water. *Giardia lamblia* protozoa are found in surface waters such as lakes and streams. Fecal runoff from livestock areas is a common vector of the disease-causing protozoa. Untreated water used for drinking or food preparation can transmit the parasites to humans. Improper personal hygiene by food service workers also can spread the infection. Giardiasis presents 1–2 weeks after infection by causing fatigue, weakness, nausea, abdominal pain, and weight loss. The illness can last for 1–2 months; however, the individual can remain infectious for several months after symptoms disappear. Giardiasis can be treated with prescription medication after positive identification of ova from stool samples (American Medical Association et al., 2004).

> **Learning Point:** Using water from approved sources and practicing good sanitation will decrease risk of giardiasis.

Parasitic Protozoa: *Cryptosporidium parvum*

Cryptosporidium parvum is a sporocyst that is resistant to many chemical disinfectants. Similar to *Giardia lamblia*, surface water can become contaminated by fecal runoff from livestock. The protozoa live in the intestinal tracts of humans and animals. Cryptosporidiosis occurs when contaminated water or uncooked food that is washed in contaminated water is consumed. The oocysts colonize the intestines, causing watery diarrhea, cramps, nausea, and slight fever within 2–10 days (CDC, 2006b). Some individuals might experience no symptoms. Cryptosporidiosis can last for several days to 3 weeks. The illness can relapse months after the symptoms disappear and can be life threatening to immunocompromised individuals (American Medical Association et al., 2004). Water testing is advisable after confirmation of cryptosporidiosis. Control methods are similar to giardiasis. The CDC reports no significant change in incidence of cryptosporidiosis in 2006 compared to the baseline period of 1996 to 1998 (CDC, 2007a).

Parasitic Protozoa: *Cyclospora cayetanensis*

Cyclosporiasis is a relatively recent parasitic illness that was first identified in 1979. Human feces are the source of infection, which can contaminate water or food. *Cyclospora* needs about 1 week after passage from the bowel to become infectious, thus it is not thought to be passed from animals to humans (American Medical Association et al., 2004). Cyclosporiasis presents as watery diarrhea, weight loss, bloating, cramps, fever, nausea, muscle aches, and fatigue about 1 week after infection. Similar to cryptosporidiosis, some individuals might experience no symptoms. Cyclosporiasis typically lasts for 1–2 weeks with relapses possible. The treatment is a combination of two antibiotics. Using water from approved sources and implementing appropriate sanitation procedures can reduce risk from cyclosporiasis (CDC, 2005h).

Parasitic Protozoa: *Toxoplasma gondii*

An estimated 60 million people in the United States are thought to be infected with the *Toxoplasma* parasite; however, a healthy immune system prevents symptoms from occurring. Immunocompromised people and pregnant women might experience serious health problems if they develop toxoplasmosis (American Medical Association et al., 2004). The parasites can be passed to humans by foods that are contaminated with cat feces or by consuming undercooked or raw meat. Cats become infected by eating wild animals and raw or undercooked meat. Pork, lamb, and venison are documented sources of the parasite. *Toxoplasma gondii* also can be spread through fecal-contaminated water. Toxoplasmosis presents as headaches, muscle aches, rash, and enlarged lymph nodes in the head and neck within 5–23 days. Symptoms frequently do not appear at the time of infection or can be confused with influenza. The illness can last for months with relapses common. Blood tests can positively identify an acute infection, which can be treated with prescription medications (CDC, 2005i).

Learning Point: The risk of contracting toxoplasmosis can be reduced by cooking meat to appropriate Food Code temperatures, avoiding cross contamination, and wearing gloves when working outdoors or cleaning litter boxes.

Table 2.1 compiles many of the pathogens that cause foodborne illnesses.

Table 2.1   Foods Implicated with Foodborne Illness

Pathogen	Poultry	Red meat	Gravy, sauces	Finfish	Shellfish	Starches	Salad	Fruit	Vegetables	Water	Dairy	Eggs
Salmonella	X	X		X	X		X	X	X		X	X
Shigella	X			X	X	X	X				X	X
Listeria monocytogenes	X	X			X	X			X		X	
Staphylococcus aureus	X	X		X	X		X				X	X
Clostridium perfringens	X	X	X			X						
Bacillus cereus		X	X	X		X	X		X			
Clostridium botulinum	X	X	X			X			X			
Escherichia coli		X					X		X	X		X
Campylobacter jejuni	X									X	X	X
Vibrio vulnificus, Vibrio parahaemolyticus					X							
Hepatitis A virus	X	X			X			X	X	X	X	
Yersinia enterocolitica		X		X	X			X	X	X		
Norovirus					X			X	X	X		
Rotavirus							X	X	X	X		
Trichinella spiralis		X										
Anisakis simplex				X	X							
Giardia lamblia								X	X	X		
Toxoplasma gondii		X										
Cryptosporidium parvum							X	X	X	X		
Cyclospora cayetanensis				X			X	X	X	X		

Source: Bad Bug Book (CDC, 2006).

Emerging Pathogens

The US food system will continue to experience new foodborne illness-causing pathogens. The incidence of new pathogens in the food supply can be attributed to several economic and demographic factors. Food imports are increasing due to the expanding global economy. Exports from developing countries with poor sanitation and inspection procedures can introduce pathogens. New foods also can harbor previously unidentified pathogens. The trend of eating fresh foods with minimal processing can increase the risk of foodborne illness. People consume more food prepared away from home, thus foregoing awareness of the sanitation practices used by the food service operation. Drugs used to treat diseases such as cancer and AIDs can make people vulnerable to foodborne pathogens. The cohort of persons over age 65 is increasing; this age group has decreased immunity. Although surveillance is improving, there is no uniform global foodborne pathogen monitoring program adopted by all nations.

In 1994, the Centers for Disease Control and Prevention implemented the Foodborne Diseases Active Surveillance Network (FoodNet) for the Emerging Infections Program to track potential foodborne enteric pathogens to the US food system (CDC, 2007a). Ten states that represent 15% of the US population are monitored for laboratory-confirmed foodborne illnesses. The number of laboratory-confirmed illnesses is divided by US Census Bureau population estimates to extrapolate the prevalence of foodborne illness. Physicians are encouraged to report specific foodborne illnesses (Table 2.2). There are several emerging pathogens that might pose a serious health threat: prions, avian flu, Brainerd diarrhea, and antimicrobial resistant *Salmonella* and *Campylobacter* (Anderson, Nelson, Baker, Rossiter, & Angulo, 2004).

Emerging Pathogens: Prions

A prion is a nonliving protein that is responsible for transmissible spongiform encephalopathy (TSE). The gene that codes for the prions is in the chromosomes of many humans and animals. TSEs occur when the prion mutates and travels through the spinal cord to the brain. The mutant prions appear to cause a chain reaction with the normal prions, leading to destruction of neurons, thus creating

Table 2.2 Foodborne Illnesses

Category of pathogen	Foodborne illness
Bacteria	Botulism
	Cholera
	Brucellosis
	Anthrax
	Enterohemorrhagic *E. coli*
	Hemolytic Uremic Syndrome
	Listeriosis
	Salmonellosis (not *S. typhi*)
	Shigellosis
	Typhoid fever (*S. typhi* and *S. paratyphi*)
Virus	Hepatitis A
Parasite	Cryptosporidiosis
	Cyclosporiasis
	Giardiasis
	Trichinellosis

Source: Compiled from http://www.fsis.usda.gov/fact_sheets/Foodborne_Illness_What_Consumers_Need_to_Know/index.asp. Retrieved September 6, 2007.

"holes" in the brain. The exact mechanism is not understood (FDA, 2006).

TSEs occur in humans as Creutzfeldt-Jakob disease (CJD), new variant Creutzfeldt-Jakob disease (nvCJD), scrapie in sheep and goats, and bovine spongiform encephalopathy (BSE) or "mad cow disease" in cattle. The incubation period can take months or years. TSEs in humans cause dementia from the deterioration of brain cells and are always fatal. Animals contract TSEs by consuming feed with nerve tissue containing the TSE. The nvCJD is a recently detected variant not related to heredity or medical procedures affecting young people. It is speculated that the nvCJD might be a result of eating beef from BSE-infected cattle. Human diagnosis for TSEs is difficult because the prions do not elicit a detectable immune response. Prions are resistant to normal sanitation practices such as heat, irradiation, and ultraviolet light. They are also resistant to antiviral and antibacterial drugs (Murano, 2003).

> **Learning Point:** Bovine spongiform encephalopathy (BSE) or "mad cow disease" is a prion.

Emerging Pathogens: Avian Influenza

Avian influenza (AI) refers to a group of influenza viruses. The virus is classified into two groups: low pathogenic avian influenza (LPAI) and highly pathogenic avian influenza (HPAI). The virulent strain HPAI H5NI is rapidly spreading among birds worldwide. Bird-to-bird transmission occurs through feces and secretions from the nose, eyes, and mouth. The onset of symptoms is rapid in birds, ranging from sneezing and coughing to decreased egg production (US Department of Agriculture [USDA], 2007).

Three major avian flu outbreaks have occurred in the United States, the latest one in 2004. All outbreaks were contained and did not spread beyond the affected region. To date no case of food-transmitted avian flu has been detected. All documented cases of human-contracted AI have been individuals who had prolonged, close contact with infected domestic birds. However, AI does not spread easily among humans (Louisiana Department of Health and Hospitals, 2007). The health concern is the mutation of avian flu to a strain that is infectious to humans. Previous major 20th century pandemics have resulted from influenza viruses that originated from birds: the "Spanish flu" of 1918, the "Asian flu" of 1957, and the "Hong Kong flu" of 1968 (Louisiana Department of Health and Hospitals, 2007). AI is controlled through normal food safety and sanitation practices, such as cooking poultry to appropriate temperatures and preventing cross contamination.

> **Learning Point:** Avian influenza (AI) is the "bird flu" disease.

Emerging Pathogens: Brainerd Diarrhea

Brainerd diarrhea is named after Brainerd, Minnesota, the location of the first documented outbreak in 1983. Symptoms present as acute watery diarrhea, cramping, fatigue, and gas. Individuals can have 10–20 episodes of watery diarrhea per day over a period of about 4 weeks. Symptoms can last up to 1 year. The etiology is unknown. Laboratory analyses of stool cultures indicate no parasites, viruses, or bacteria present. Untreated well water and raw milk have been associated with outbreaks. The disease appears to be self-limiting, with no recommended treatment (CDC, 2005j).

Resources

Table 2.3 lists agencies that assist with foodborne illness and their Web sites.

Chapter Summary

Foodborne illness-causing pathogens include bacteria, viruses, and parasites. The acronym "FAT TOM" (food, acidity, time, temperature, oxygen, and moisture) describes the general conditions that favor growth of foodborne pathogens. Foodborne illnesses most often result from time–temperature abuse, cross contamination, and poor personal hygiene. Although the US food system is one of the safest in the world, absolute safety is not possible. Human error, intentional contamination, and mutation of pathogenic organisms all pose risk of foodborne illness. Microorganisms can never be eliminated from the environment; thus appropriate sanitation measures will always be necessary. Specific food safety issues and related control measures will be described in the following chapters.

Issues to Debate

1. Discuss whether humans or the food itself poses a major risk to food safety.
2. Describe the conditions that encourage foodborne infections, intoxications, and intoxifications.
3. In the past 100 years, illnesses such as typhoid fever and botulism were more common than they are now. Explain the environmental changes that have decreased the incidence of some foodborne illnesses and increased the incidence of others.
4. Is the US population more or less vulnerable to foodborne illness-causing pathogens?

Table 2.3 Federal Agencies and Web Sites with Food Safety Responsibilities

Agency	Unit	Mission	URL
US Department of Agriculture (USDA)	Animal and Plant Health Inspection Service (APHIS)	Protects and promotes US agricultural health	USDA: http://www.usda.gov APHIS: http://aphis.usda.gov
	Food Safety and Inspection Service (FSIS)	Ensures that the nation's commercial supply of meat, poultry, and egg products is safe, wholesome, and correctly labeled and packaged	http://www.fsis.usda.gov
	Agricultural Research Service (ARS), National Animal Disease Center (NADC)	Conducts research on animal health and food safety problems	http://www.nadc.ars.usda.gov
	ARS, Poultry Processing Research Unit	Conducts research on factors affecting poultry meat quality and microbiological safety	http://ppmq.ars.usda.gov
Department of Commerce (USDC)	National Oceanic and Atmospheric Administration (NOAA)	Administers National Seafood Inspection Program (NSIP), which offers seafood inspection,	USDC: http://www.commerce.gov NOAA: http://www.noaa.gov

		grading, certification, and other services to the seafood industry (voluntary, fee-for-service)	NSIP: http://seafood.nmfs.noaa.gov
US Department of Health and Human Services (HHS)	Centers for Disease Control and Prevention (CDC)	Tracks foodborne illness incidents and outbreaks; provides data and information to the other food safety agencies	HHS: http://www.os.dhhs.gov CDC: http://www.cdc.gov
	Food and Drug Administration (FDA)	Approves food and drugs for widespread use; its Center for Food Safety and Applied Nutrition (CFSAN) ensures that food is safe, nutritious, and wholesome	FDA: http://www.fda.gov CFSAN: http://vm.cfsan.fda.gov/list.html
Department of Homeland Security (DHS)	Customs and Border Protection (CBP)	Inspects agricultural goods arriving in the United States at ports and borders	DHS: http://www.dhs.gov/dhspublic/ CBP: http://www.customs.ustreas.gov CBP Agriculture Specialist Fact Sheet:

(continues)

Table 2.3 Federal Agencies and Web Sites with Food Safety Responsibilities *(continued)*

Agency	Unit	Mission	URL
			http://www.cbp.gov/ linkhandler/cgov/newsroom/ fact_sheets/printer_fact_ sheets/agriculture.ctt/ agriculture.pdf
Department of Treasury	Bureau of Alcohol, Tobacco, Firearms and Explosives	Regulates qualification and operations of distilleries, wineries, breweries, importers, and wholesalers	Treasury: http://www.ustreas.gov ATF: http://www.atf.gov
Federal Trade Commission	Bureau of Consumer Protection (BCP); Division of Advertising Practices (DAP); Division of Consumer Protection (DCP); Division of Enforcement (DE)	Protects consumers against unfair, deceptive, or fraudulent practices; protects consumers from deceptive and unsubstantiated advertising (advertising claims for food, particularly those relating to nutritional or health benefits of foods); conducts law enforcement activities to protect consumers	FTC: http://www.ftc.gov BCP: http://www.ftc.gov/bcp/ bcp.htm DAP: http://www.ftc.gov/bcp/ bcpap.htm DE: http://www.ftc.gov/bcp/ bcpenf.htm

References

American Medical Association, American Nurses Association, Centers for Disease Control, Center for Food Safety and Applied Nutrition, Food Safety and Inspection Service. (2004). *Foodborne illnesses table: Parasitic agents.* Retrieved July 1, 2007, from http://www.cfsan.fda.gov/~pat.htm

Anderson, A. D., Nelson, M., Baker, N. L., Rossiter, S., & Angulo, F. J. (2004). *Public health consequences of use of antimicrobial agents in agriculture. Risk management strategies, monitoring and surveillance.* Retrieved July 2, 2007, from http://www.cdc.gov/enterics/2_a_anderson_2003.pdf.

Brown, A. (2005). Food safety. In *Understanding food* (2nd ed.). Belmont, CA: Wadsworth/Thomson Learning.

Centers for Disease Control. (2005a, October 12). *Salmonellosis.* Retrieved July 2, 2007, from http://www.cdc.gov/ncidod/dbmd/diseaseinfo/salmonellosis_g.htm

Centers for Disease Control. (2005b, October 12). *Shigellosis.* Retrieved July 2, 2007, from http://www.cdc.gov/ncidod/dbmd/diseaseinfo/shigellosis_g.htm

Centers for Disease Control. (2005c, October 12). *Botulism.* Retrieved July 1, 2007, from http://www.cdc.gov/ncidod/dbmd/diseaseinfo/botulism_g.htm

Centers for Disease Control. (2005d, October 12). *Vibrio parahaemolyticus.* Retrieved July 2, 2007, from http://www.cdc.gov/ncidod/dbmd/diseaseinfo/vibrioparahaemolyticus_g.htm

Centers for Disease Control. (2005e, October 12). *Vibrio vulnificus.* Retrieved July 2, 2007, from http://www.cdc.gov/ncidod/dbmd/diseaseinfo/vibriovulnificus_g.htm

Centers for Disease Control. (2005f, October 12). *Norovirus in Healthcare Facilities—Fact Sheet.* Retrieved July 2, 2007, from http://www.cdc.gov/ncidod/dvrd/revb/gastro/norovirus.htm

Centers for Disease Control. (2005g, October 12). *Trichinellosis fact sheet for the general public.* Retrieved July 1, 2007, from http://www.cdc.gov/ncidod/dpd/parasites/trichinosis/factsht_trichinosis.htm

Centers for Disease Control. (2005h, October 12). *Cyclospora infection fact sheet.* Retrieved July 1, 2007, from http://www.cdc.gov/ncidod/dpd/parasites/cyclospora/factsht_cyclospora.htm

Centers for Disease Control. (2005i, October 12). *Toxoplasmosis fact sheet.* Retrieved July 2, 2007, from http://www.cdc.gov/ncidod/dpd/parasites/toxoplasmosis/factsht_toxoplasmosis.htm

Centers for Disease Control. (2005j, October 5). *Brainerd diarrhea.* Retrieved July 2, 2007, from http://www.cdc.gov/ncidod/dbmd/diseaseinfo/brainerddiarrhea_g.htm

Centers for Disease Control. (2006a, December 6). *Escherichia coli O157:H7.* Retrieved July 2, 2007, from http://www.cdc.gov/ncidod/dbmd/diseaseinfo/escherichiacoli_g.htm

Centers for Disease Control. (2006b, August 3). *Viral gastroenteritis.* Retrieved July 2, 2007, from http://www.cdc.gov/ncidod/dvrd/revb/ gastro/faq.htm

Centers for Disease Control. (2007a). Preliminary FoodNet data on the incidence of infection with pathogens transmitted commonly through food— 10 states, 2006. *Mortality and Morbidity Weekly Report, 56*(14), 336–339. Retrieved July 2, 2007, from http://www.cdc.gov/mmwr/ preview/mmwrhtml/mm5614a4.htm

Centers for Disease Control. (2007b, March 26). *About Rotavirus.* Retrieved July 2, 2007, from http://www.cdc.gov/rotavirus/about_rotavirus.htm

Fiore, A. E. (2004). Hepatitis A transmitted by food. *Clinical Infectious Diseases, 38*:705–515.

Food and Drug Administration. (2007a, June 12). *Lettuce safety initiative.* Retrieved July 2, 2007, from http://www.cfsan.fda.gov/~dms/ lettsafe.html

Food and Drug Administration. (2007b, June 12). *Tomato safety initiative.* Retrieved July 2, 2007, from http://www.cfsan.fda.gov/~dms/ tomsafe.html

Food and Drug Administration, Center for Food Safety and Applied Nutrition. (2005). *FDA food code.* Retrieved July 1, 2007, from http:// www.cfsan.fda.gov/~dms/foodcode.html

Food and Drug Administration, Center for Food Safety and Applied Nutrition. (2006, April 25). *Foodborne pathogenic microorganisms and natural toxins handbook (Bad bug book).* Retrieved July 1, 2007, from http:// vm.cfsan.fda.gov/~mow/intro.html

Frenzen, P. D., Drake A., & Angulo, F. J. (2005). Economic cost of illness due to *Escherichia coli* O157:H7 infections in the United States. *Journal of Food Protection, 68*(12), 2623–2630.

Louisiana Department of Health and Hospitals, Center for Community Preparedness. (2007). *How you can be prepared for a flu pandemic* [Brochure]. South Deerfield, MA: Channing Bete Company.

Mead, P. S., Slutsker, L., Dietz, V., McCaig, L. F., Bresee, J. S., Shapiro, C., et al. (1999). Food-related illness and death in the United States. *Emerging Infectious Diseases, 5*(5), 605–617.

Murano, P. (2003). Food safety. In *Understanding food science and technology.* Belmont, CA: Thomson Wadsworth.

National Restaurant Association Educational Foundation. (2005). *Servsafe coursebook* (4th ed.). Chicago: Author.

Samuel, M. C., Vugia, D. J., Shallow, S., Marcus, R., Segler, S., & McGivern, T. (2004). Epidemiology of sporadic campylobacter infection in the United States and declining trend in incidence, FoodNet 1996–1999. *Clinical Infectious Diseases, 38*(Suppl 3), S165–174.

US Department of Agriculture. (2007, March). *Questions and answers: Avian influenza* (Release No. 0458.05). Retrieved July 2, 2007, from http:// www.usda.gov/wps/portal/!ut/p/_s.7_0_1RD.htm

CHAPTER 3

SAFETY ISSUES IN THE US FOOD SYSTEM

Bonnie L. Gerald, PhD, DTR

Chapter Objectives

After reading the chapter and reflecting on the contents, you should be able to:

1. Define the relationship between each part of the food system and how the parts work as a system.
2. Differentiate the implications of foodborne illness-causing pathogens in one part of the food system and the subsequent impact to other parts of the food system.
3. Articulate the potential food safety hazards present in soil, water, plants, and animals.
4. Describe the potential food safety hazards during harvest, processing, and distribution of food.
5. Assess the magnitude of risk present in each part of the food system.

Key Terms

biological toxins: Poisonous substances produced by living cells or organisms.
food toxicology: The study of the adverse effects and/or poisoning of food substances on living organisms.
mycotoxins: A poisonous substance produced by a fungus organism, which includes some mushrooms, molds, and yeast.
neurotoxications: Chemicals in foods that can cause profuse sweating, excitement, depression, coma, convulsions, and hallucinations.

Introduction

The US food system is considered to be one of the safest in the world. The US food production and distribution system is diverse, extensive, and readily accessible. However, changing demographic and economic factors present numerous challenges to the food system. The open food system is susceptible to pathogens and toxins from natural and deliberate processes (Agricultural Research Service [ARS], 2006a). This chapter will provide background on the elements of the food system: soil, water, animals, plants, production, and processing. It is necessary to understand the interrelationship of the parts of the food system prior to identifying and assessing hazards present in the US food system.

The Food System: Climate

Modern agricultural practices have made it possible to produce food in areas previously unsuitable for agriculture production. For example, we can grow citrus in the desert and produce over 200 bushels of corn per acre. The result has been increased variety and quantity of foods available. However, modern technology has not changed fundamental aspects of food production. Adequate water, sunlight, and temperatures remain essential agricultural inputs. Climate has a pivotal role in determining which plants and animals will thrive in a given area. For example, temperate regions that receive 35–45 inches of rainfall annually can produce crops with minimal irrigation. Areas with mild winters and rainfall less than 35 inches annually support cattle that are acclimated to these conditions. For example, cattle raised in the Florida panhandle will have a different genetic background than cattle raised in the Nebraska sand hills. Cattle raised in the Nebraska sand hills must have the ability to survive a wide temperature range (−20°F to over 100°F). Florida ranchers will raise cattle with the ability to tolerate extended periods of

Learning Point: Producing food in areas not previously associated with the particular food (i.e., growing citrus crops in the desert) can result in safety hazards not seen in food raised in its usual environment.

hot, dry weather. Climate also determines the types of microorganisms that are capable of surviving in a particular environment.

The Food System: Soil

Soil is the second major determinant of the types of foods produced in a specific area. Soil is comprised of organic matter, minerals, gas, and water. It is the boundary between air, plants (upper), and parent material (lower). The soil thickness varies, but it generally extends 200 cm below the soil surface (Natural Resource Conservation Service [NRCS], 2006a). Factors responsible for soil formation are its parent material, climate, topography, biological factors, and time (NRCS, 2006b). Soils are not static; they evolve continuously, responding to natural and man-made changes in the environment. For example, soil pH can change due to agricultural runoff or as a result of natural weathering. The pH change will facilitate growth of some microorganisms over others, thus changing the potential safety hazard. The application of organic fertilizers can facilitate pathogen growth. Infusions (compost tea) prepared from composted fruits and vegetables can support *E. coli* O157:H7 and *Salmonella* if it is supplemented with nutrients. The compost tea is used to control foliar and root diseases of fresh produce (Millner & Ingram, 2007).

The Food System: Water

Water is essential for all living things. Water used for domestic purposes must be treated to meet requirements of the Safe Drinking Water Act. Treatment is required for domestic water whether it originates from surface or groundwater sources. Several microorganisms are resistant to chlorine; alternative methods such as UV radiation must be used to kill the pathogens. The quality of water for agricultural production is not regulated by the government. The treatment of groundwater depends on the depth of the water-bearing material (aquifer). Unless it is contaminated by human activity, water from deep wells will not have high bacterial or protozoa content.

Surface water from reservoirs, lakes, and rivers can contain high levels of harmful microorganisms. The microorganisms can result from agricultural runoff, untreated sewage, or decaying organic matter in the body of water. This is called "nonpoint pollution" because the source of contamination is not easily identified. Toxins from manufacturing processes also can be discharged into surface water. This is an example of "point pollution" because the contamination can be traced to its source. Excess irrigation water can be held in pits for reuse on crops. This water can be contaminated by uncomposted manure or other agricultural runoff. The reused water can seep into the aquifer, thus contaminating the groundwater. Another potential source of microbial contamination is broken water pipes that allow microorganisms that are present in the soil to enter the water supply. This situation was responsible for the 1993 cryptosporidiosis outbreak in Milwaukee.

> **Learning Point:** It is estimated that 25% to 50% of water in municipal water systems is lost through broken water lines.

The Food System: Animals and Fish

Animals are a major source of foodborne illness-causing pathogens. Both domestic and wild animals are sources of bacteria, viruses, and parasites. Microorganisms living in the animals' intestines are excreted in the feces. The fecal matter can contaminate water and soil that is used for crop production. Runoff containing fecal matter can contaminate water sources. Uncomposted manure that is used as fertilizer also can contaminate crops and soils. Intestinal contents can contact meat during processing, thus contaminating the meat.

> **Learning Point:** Parasites living in animal or fish muscles can be transmitted to humans if not cooked to the appropriate temperature.

Poultry also are sources of bacteria, viruses, and parasites. Their intestines are a source of bacterial contamination during processing. *Salmonella* also is common on the surface of chicken and turkey carcasses. Fecal bacteria can be transmitted from the hen's cloaca to its eggs. The egg shell is porous; bacteria can pass through the shell if the eggs are not washed completely during processing. Bird viruses have mutated into forms that are harmful to humans. Chapter 2 describes the avian flu virus and its potential impact to human health.

Antibiotics have been added to animal feed and water to prevent or eliminate harmful bacteria. There are four general categories of animal antibiotics:

1. Aminoglycosides, such as streptomycin, interfere with protein synthesis of bacteria. The aminoglycosides are used for *Brucella*, *Salmonella*, *Klebsiella*, *Shigella*, and *Mycobacterium*.
2. Chloramphenicol inhibits bacterial cell wall synthesis and is used for treating salmonellosis, brucellosis, and bacterial pneumonia.
3. Macrolides are administered when bacteria are resistant to other antibiotics. It functions as a bacterial growth inhibitor. The macrolide erythromycin has raised concerns about increased bacterial resistance when the drug is used. Bacterial resistance to penicillin drugs also has been documented.
4. Sulfa drugs, such as tetracycline, can pass to the milk of dairy cows. Cases of human sensitivity to sulfa drugs and chloramphenicol have been documented (Murano, 2003a).

Scientists believe that antibiotic resistance in humans is linked to antibiotic resistance in animals. Bacteria living in animals' intestines become resistant to the antibiotics in their feed and water. The resistant pathogenic bacteria are shed in animal feces, which then go into lakes, rivers, and soil. These bacteria also can be present on meat and milk from the affected animals. Overuse of human antibiotics can contribute to bacterial resistance. The resistant bacteria are shed in human feces and can spread by sewage contacting the environment (Murano, 2003a). For example, *Salmonella enterica* serotype Typhimurium phage type DT 104, an antibiotic-resistant virulent strain of *Salmonella*, has been detected in ground retail meat (Carlson, Wu, & Frana, 2003).

Fish and shellfish can ingest species of toxic algae that grow in bays and estuaries. The algal blooms are cyclical; however, no one can predict where the toxic algae concentrations will occur. Fish and shellfish that are harvested from areas with toxic algae will pass the toxins to humans when the contaminated seafood is consumed. For example, ciguatera toxin produced by the dinoflagellate *Gambierdiscus toxicus* accumulates in the bodies of predatory reef fish, such as grouper, mackerel, snapper, amberjack, and barracuda (Food and

Drug Administration [FDA], 2006a). The toxin cannot be destroyed by cooking or freezing, and it results in ciguatera poisoning. The symptoms are nausea, vomiting, itching, hot and cold flashes, and temporary blindness. Recovery can take weeks or months. Shellfish also can be contaminated with toxins produced by planktonic algae. Red tide, a reddish marine alga, produces toxins that can contaminate shellfish.

There are four types of shellfish toxins:

1. Paralytic
2. Diarrheic
3. Neurotoxic
4. Amnesic

Learning Point: Seafood toxins are tasteless and odorless and cannot be destroyed by cooking or freezing. The most effective control method is to purchase fish and shellfish only from approved sources (FDA, 2006b).

The Food System: Plants

Plants also can be sources of foodborne illness-causing pathogens. Some plants naturally produce toxins that should be avoided by humans: rhubarb leaves, jimsonweed, and water hyacinth roots. Other plants, such as kidney beans and fava beans, are toxic until thoroughly cooked. Phytohemagglutinin is the toxic compound that must be destroyed by adequate cooking of kidney and fava beans. Honey that is produced from the nectar of some species of rhododendrons is toxic to humans. Grayanotoxins in the honey can interfere with cardiac functioning and blood pressure.

Fruits and vegetables can become contaminated with pathogens as a result of being grown in soils containing fecal matter or water containing bacteria, viruses, or parasites. Outbreaks of foodborne illness from alfalfa sprouts (*E. coli*), tomatoes (*Salmonella*), and spinach (*E. coli*) are examples of food that is contaminated by pathogens in the soil and water. Plants take water and nutrients from the soil, and then they are transported by the plant's vascular system to the leaves and fruit. Bacteria also can be transported with the water and nutrients to edible parts of the plant. Outbreaks of salmonellosis from sliced melons are examples of bacteria that enter the plant through the root system (National Restaurant Association Educational Foundation [NRAEF], 2005a).

The Food System: Fungi

Fungi include mushrooms, yeasts, and molds. Numerous varieties of fungi naturally produce toxins. Mushrooms, particularly wild mushrooms, are the cause of most of the reported intoxications. The toxin-producing mushrooms are widespread, ranging from suburban lawns to the wilderness. Because of the difficulty in identifying mushroom species, illnesses from consuming mushrooms are identified by the type of toxin produced. Mushroom toxins are categorized by their effect: gastrointestinal irritants, neurotoxins, protoplasms, and disulfiram-like intoxications.

> **Learning Point:** Toxins cannot be destroyed by cooking or freezing.

Gastrointestinal Irritants

Gastrointestinal irritants are the mildest form of intoxication. Symptoms present as nausea, vomiting, diarrhea, and abdominal cramps. The intoxication has a rapid onset, is short-lived, and is rarely fatal. The Green Gill, Gray Pinkgill, Early False Morel, and Tigertop are examples of gastrointestinal irritant-producing toxins (FDA, 2006c).

Neurotoxins

Mushrooms that contain neurotoxins can cause profuse sweating, excitement, depression, coma, convulsions, and hallucinations. Three groups of neurotoxins are responsible for most of the neurotoxications. Muscarine toxin is characterized by profuse sweating and occasional hallucinations. The onset is rapid, within 15–30 minutes of consumption, and usually subsides within 2 hours. *Inocybe* and *Clitocybe* are species that are associated with muscarine poisoning. Ibotenic acid/muscimol intoxication presents as drowsiness or dizziness, followed by periods of hyperactivity. Symptoms occur 1–2 hours after ingestion and are gone within several hours. Panthercap and Fly Agaric mushrooms (*Amanita* species) produce these two toxins. Psilocybin intoxication symptoms appear to be similar to alcohol intoxication; however, drowsiness does not occur. Hallucinations also can occur with the *Psilocybe* genera. Intoxication onset occurs fairly rapidly after ingestion and lasts about 2 hours. Some Native American tribes have used the *Psilocybe* mushroom as part of their religious practice (FDA, 2006d).

Protoplasms

Mushrooms that produce protoplasmic toxin cause the most damage and can be fatal when eaten. If untreated for 60 or more hours after ingestion, victims of protoplasmic intoxication have a 50% to 90% fatality rate. The protoplasmic toxins are characterized by a latency period, acute symptoms, and cellular destruction, which can lead to organ failure. There are three types of protoplasmic toxins: amatoxins, hydrazines, and orellanine. Amatoxins have a latency period of 6–15 hours, followed by vomiting, watery diarrhea, and abdominal pain. The acute symptoms might abate; however, the toxin causes liver, kidney, skeletal, and cardiac damage, leading to convulsions and coma. Survivors have enlarged livers. Death Cap, Destroying Angel, and Autumn Skullcap are examples of the amanitine-producing mushrooms. Hydrazines are produced by the False Morel species (*Gyromitra*). Symptoms are similar to amanitine intoxication but are less severe and have a lower fatality rate. Orellanine toxin has a long latency period of 3–14 days, followed by extreme thirst and excessive urination. Nausea, chills, headache, and muscular pain are acute symptoms, followed by liver, intestinal, and renal damage. The mortality rate is approximately 15%, resulting from renal failure. The Sorrel Webcap mushroom (*Cortinarius orellanus*) produces the orellanine toxin (FDA, 2006e).

Disulfiram-Like Intoxications

The Inky Cap (*Coprinus atrimentarius*) mushroom is harmless when it is not consumed with alcohol. The amino acid coprine in the mushroom inhibits alcohol metabolism, resulting in nausea, vomiting, flushing, and headache if consumed within 72 hours of drinking alcohol. Symptoms last for several hours but do not appear to cause long-term damage (FDA, 2006f).

Aflatoxin

Aflatoxins are produced by strains of *Aspergillus flavus* and *A. parasiticus*. The fungi grow on nuts and grains under heat and drought conditions. Aflatoxins have been detected on cottonseed, corn, peanuts, tree nuts, and other oilseeds. Aflatoxicosis affects the liver in animals. The toxin can be excreted in milk and urine of dairy cattle. The aflatoxin strain B1 is a known carcinogen in birds, fish, rodents, and nonhuman primates. Human cases have been documented in Kenya and India, although the extent of human aflatoxicosis is unknown (FDA, 2006g).

Yeasts and Molds

Yeasts and molds are generally considered to be spoilage microorganisms. However, some yeasts and molds are a normal part of food production. Examples are the yeast strain *Saccharomyces cerevisiae*, which produces alcohol from grain, and the mold *Penicillium roqueforti*, which is added during cheese ripening to produce blue cheese.

Spoiled food is characterized by off-odors, off-flavors, changed color, or sliminess. Yeasts can metabolize carbohydrates in grains, fruits, and vegetables if warm, moist conditions are present. Molds also can metabolize carbohydrates in fruits and vegetables. *Penicillium citrinum* degrades pectin in citrus fruits, causing soft rot. Cellulose is broken down by the molds *Aspergillus* and *Penicillium*, resulting in softening of vegetables. Meat pigments can be affected by mold. Color changes result from growth of *Cladosporium herbarum* (black spots), *Sporotrichum* (white spots), and *Thamnidium* (fuzzy growth) (Murano, 2003b).

Several grain molds are capable of causing foodborne illness. *Claviceps purpurea* (ergot mold) grows on wheat, rye, barley, and oats under cool, damp conditions. If the harvested grain has more than 0.3% *Claviceps* by weight, it is considered to be ergoty. The mold is removed by normal milling processes but can contaminate feed grains. Gangrenous ergotism causes loss of circulation in the feet and hands. Convulsive ergotism causes hallucinations and convulsions.

Fusarium molds can grow under freezing temperatures, affecting oats, barley, rye, and wheat (Glenn, 2003). Consumption of the *Fusarium* toxin trichothecene can cause alimentary toxic aleukia. After the acute stage of nausea, vomiting, and cramps, a latent stage causes damage to the bone marrow, which leads to other complications such as leukemia and pneumonia. *F. moniliforme* has been linked to esophageal cancer. *Fusarium* intoxications are relatively uncommon, but the mortality rates can be as high as 80% (Murano, 2003c). The virulence of trichothecene toxins is variable worldwide due to the complex genetic makeup of *F. graminearum* populations (McCormick & Desjardins, 2006).

Naturally occurring fungi can produce harmful mycotoxins. Mushroom intoxications can be avoided by purchasing mushrooms only from approved sources. Spoilage microorganisms generally leave physical clues that the food is unfit to eat. Assays for detection of *Fusarium*, aflatoxins, *Claviceps*, and other mycotoxins are being developed (Glenn, 2003; Gao, Luo, & Lee, 2004; ARS, 2006b).

The Food System: Raw Ingredient to Food

Foodborne illness-causing pathogens can be introduced at the harvest, processing, and distribution phases of any food. Using good agricultural practices (GAP) and good manufacturing processes (GMP) can prevent or minimize hazards.

Harvesting

Fresh produce should be transported as quickly as possible to the processing center. Reducing field heat decreases one of the factors necessary for pathogen growth in addition to preserving nutritional quality. Workers should have access to clean water and sanitary facilities to help prevent bacterial contamination.

Fish and shellfish should be placed in cold storage immediately. Fish such as tuna, mackerel, mahi-mahi, and marlin can cause histamine poisoning if they are time–temperature abused during harvest and processing. The bacteria naturally present on the fish produce a histamine toxin that cannot be destroyed by cooking or freezing. Symptoms include a burning sensation in the mouth, flushing, sweating, headache, and nausea (NRAEF, 2005b).

Food is withheld from animals generally 12–24 hours prior to slaughter. The purpose is to empty the intestines as much as possible, thus decreasing the risk of fecal contamination during processing.

Processing

GMPs minimize food contact with contaminated soil, air, and water. Food contact surfaces must be cleaned and sanitized to prevent cross contamination. Common sanitizers used on equipment are chlorine, iodine, quaternary ammonium, and organic acids. Chemicals used to process food also can contaminate it. Potential chemical toxicants are cleaners, sanitizers, pesticides, lubricants, and paints. Refrigeration (39°F to 44°F) and freezing (0°F to −10°F) temperatures are the most widely used methods to inhibit bacterial growth. Cold temperatures slow pathogenic and spoilage microbial growth but do not stop it. Bacteriostatic methods do not kill pathogens but prevent them from growing. Examples include smoking, drying, and the preservatives sulfite and sodium nitrite. Heat is considered to be a bactericidal method because it kills bacterial cells. Food with high fat content or that has low moisture can decrease heat's effectiveness as a bacteriocide. Heat-resistant microorganisms, such as bacterial spores and gram-positive bacteria, can survive temperatures that kill other biological hazards. Chemical bacteriocides have been used on fresh produce. Some bacteria have become resistant to the chemicals, most notably on honeydew melons and apples (Leverctz et al., 2003). It is impossible to eliminate all pathogens when producing food. GMPs and standard sanitation operating procedures (SSOP) must be implemented in all food processing facilities to minimize biological and chemical hazards.

Transport and Distribution

Time–temperature control is essential for moving food through the system. Foods can be monitored using supply chain technology. A numeric 14 digit coding system can be used to identify batches of products or single items. The codes make possible the use of radio frequency identification, bar coding, and data synchronization to track foods from supplier to buyer. The majority of food producers use the coding technology. An exception is the produce sector, which does increase the risk of pathogen-containing food being widely distributed before a problem is documented (Reynolds, 2007). Transport vehicles must be capable of maintaining the appropriate temperature for the food item. Food temperatures should be checked at each delivery point in the supply chain. Foods exceeding their safe temperature limits or that have had their integrity compromised should be returned for credit.

Receiving and Storage

Foods should be purchased from approved sources. An approved source is defined as an organization that has been inspected and meets all local, state, and federal laws. After checking the condition of the food, it should be moved immediately to storage. Delivery times should be scheduled when staff is available to receive the items. This decreases the opportunity for contamination by pests and vermin.

The refrigerator air temperature must be kept at least 2°F lower than the desired temperature. If foods need storage at 40°F, then the air temperature should measure 38°F at the warmest point in the storage unit, usually next to the door. Freezers should be kept at 0°F or lower. Thermometers should be installed next to the doors for ease of monitoring. Temperatures should be checked at least once per shift. Dry storage should be at least 6 inches from the floor at a temperature range of 50°F to 70°F (NRAEF, 2005c). A relative humidity of 50% to 60% in the storeroom should be maintained.

Food Production and Service

Whether prepared at home or away from home, production and service is the last step in the food system. Foodborne illness can still occur, even if the food has been properly handled up to the point of production. The Centers for Disease Control and Prevention (CDC) estimates that 80% of foodborne illnesses can be traced to food that is prepared outside the home, while about 20% can be attributed to home preparation (CDC, 2007). These statistics are evidence that much work needs to be done to educate food service employees and consumers. This chapter has described many potential sources of natural and man-made contaminants in the food supply. The following chapters will discuss the food safety legal environment and describe methods used to control potential sources of foodborne illness in the food system.

> **Learning Point:** The three most common causes of foodborne illness are time–temperature abuse, cross contamination, and poor personal hygiene. All of these factors can be controlled.

Chapter Summary

Food safety is a farm-to-fork continuum. The types of pathogens in the food system are determined by climate, soil, and water where the plants or animals are raised. Microorganisms can be passed from the soil and water to plants and animals. Animals often are biological sources of contamination of soil and water. Some toxins are naturally generated by plants, animals, and fungi. Chemical intoxications are unintentional results of growing and processing food. Harvesting and processing can introduce biological pathogens to the food by unsanitary conditions. Time–temperature abuse, cross contamination, and poor personal hygiene are food safety issues as it moves from the processor to the consumer.

Issues to Debate

1. There are numerous opportunities for food to become unsafe as it moves through the food system. Identify one part of the system that presents the greatest threat to consumers, in your opinion.
2. Describe the path of a bacterial pathogen from farm to fork for: cantaloupe, ground beef, or corn.
3. In your opinion, how many of the food safety issues in the food system today are the result of human activities? How many are the result of natural processes?
4. Which of the bacterial pathogens appears to be the most resistant or viable as they travel through the food system, in your opinion?
5. Are antibiotics administered too frequently to animals and humans? Discuss the potential consequences if antibiotics are not routinely given to animals or humans, except in the most extreme cases.

Web Sites

The Centers for Disease Control Weekly Morbidity and Mortality
Report
http://www.cdc.gov/mmwr/

The Centers for Disease Control data for age-specific trends and
pathogen trends
http://www.cdc.gov/foodnet

The Center for Food Safety and Applied Nutrition
http://www.cfsan.fda.gov

International Association for Food Protection
www.foodprotection.org

National Environmental Health Association
www.neha.org

American Society for Microbiology
www.asm.org

The Mushroom Council
www.mushroomcouncil.com

National Center for Preparedness, Detection, and Control of Infectious Diseases
www.cdc.gov/ncpdcid

Compendium of Fish and Fishery Product Processes, Hazards, and
Controls
http://seafood.ucdavis.edu/haccp/compendium/compend.htm

FoodSafety Magazine
www.foodsafetymagazine.com

References

Agricultural Research Service. (2006a). Executive summary. *National pro-
    gram 108: Food safety 2006 annual report.* Beltsville, MD: Author. Re-
    trieved July 13, 2007, from http://www.ars.usda.gov/sp2UserFiles/
    Program/108/2006reportforweb.pdf
Agricultural Research Service. (2006b). Mycotoxin methods developed to make
    toxin identification easier. *National program 108: Food safety 2006*

annual report. Beltsville, MD: Author. Retrieved July 13, 2007, from
   http://www.ars.usda.gov/sp2UserFiles/Program/108/2006reportforweb.pdf
Carlson, S., Wu, M., & Frana, T. (2003). Multiple antibiotic resistance and
   virulence of *Salmonella enterica* serotype Typhimurium phage type DT
   104. In R. E. Isaacson & M. E. Torrence (Eds.), *Current topics in food
   safety and animal agriculture* (pp. 123–129). Ames, IA: Iowa State University Press.
Centers for Disease Control. (2007). Preliminary FoodNet data on the incidence of infection with pathogens transmitted commonly through food—
   10 states, 2006. *Mortality and Morbidity Weekly Report, 56*(14),
   336–339. Retrieved July 2, 2007, from http://www.cdc.gov/mmwr/
   preview/mmwrhtml/mm5614a4.htm
Food and Drug Administration. (2006a). Ciguatera. In *Foodborne pathogenic
   microorganisms and natural toxins handbook* (*Bad bug book*) (pp. 165–166).
   Retrieved July 12, 2007, from http://vm.cfsan.fda.gov/~mow/intro.html
Food and Drug Administration. (2006b). Various shellfish-associated toxins.
   In *Foodborne pathogenic microorganisms and natural toxins handbook*
   (*Bad bug book*) (pp. 170–173). Retrieved July 12, 2007, from http://
   vm.cfsan.fda.gov/~mow/intro.html
Food and Drug Administration. (2006c). Gastrointestinal irritants. In *Foodborne pathogenic microorganisms and natural toxins handbook* (*Bad bug
   book*) (p. 201). Retrieved July 12, 2007, from http://vm.cfsan.fda.gov/
   ~mow/intro.html
Food and Drug Administration. (2006d). Neurotoxins. In *Foodborne pathogenic microorganisms and natural toxins handbook* (*Bad bug book*)
   (pp. 200–201). Retrieved July 12, 2007, from http://vm.cfsan.fda.gov/
   ~mow/intro.html
Food and Drug Administration. (2006e). Protoplasmic poisons. In *Foodborne
   pathogenic microorganisms and natural toxins handbook* (*Bad bug book*)
   (pp. 198–199). Retrieved July 12, 2007, from http://vm.cfsan.fda.gov/
   ~mow/intro.html
Food and Drug Administration. (2006f). Disulfiram-like poisoning. In *Foodborne pathogenic microorganisms and natural toxins handbook* (*Bad bug
   book*) (pp. 201–202). Retrieved July 12, 2007, from http://vm.cfsan.fda.gov/
   ~mow/intro.html
Food and Drug Administration. (2006g). Aflatoxins. In *Foodborne pathogenic
   microorganisms and natural toxins handbook* (*Bad bug book*) (pp. 216–220).
   Retrieved July 12, 2007, from http://vm.cfsan.fda.gov/~mow/intro.html
Gao, B., Luo, M., & Lee, D. (2004, May). Functional genomic approach to
   eliminate aflatoxin contamination in corn [Abstract]. *Proceedings of the
   15th International Plant Protection Congress*, Beijing, China.
Glenn, A. (2003). Fumonisin contamination of corn and development of cellular, biological, and environmental control strategies. *Mycopathologia,
   155*, 30–32.
Leveretz, B., Conway, W., Camp, M., Janisiewicz, W., Abuladze, T., Saftner,
   R., et al. (2003). Biocontrol of *Listeria monocytogenes* on fresh-cut

produce by combining bacteriophages and a bacteriocin. *Applied and Environmental Microbiology, 69*, 4519–4526.

McCormick, S., & Desjardins, A. (2006, June). Emerging mycotoxin issues [Abstract]. *47th Annual Dry Corn Milling Proceedings*, 10.

Millner, P., & Ingram, D. (2007). Growth and survival of *Escherichia coli* O157:H7 and *Salmonella enteritidis* in compost tea. *Journal of Food Protection, 70*, 828–834.

Murano, P. S. (2003a). Food toxicology. In *Understanding food science and technology* (pp. 344–345). Belmont, CA: Wadsworth.

Murano, P. S. (2003b). Food microbiology and fermentation. In *Understanding food science and technology* (pp. 291–292). Belmont, CA: Wadsworth.

Murano, P. S. (2003c). Food safety. In *Understanding food science and technology* (pp. 311–312). Belmont, CA: Wadsworth.

National Restaurant Association Educational Foundation. (2005a). The microworld. In *Servsafe coursebook* (4th ed.) (pp. 2-12–2-15). Chicago: Author.

National Restaurant Association Educational Foundation. (2005b). Contamination, food allergens, and foodborne illness. In *Servsafe coursebook* (4th ed.) (pp. 3-5–3-4). Chicago: Author.

National Restaurant Association Educational Foundation. (2005c). The flow of food: Storage. In *Servsafe coursebook* (4th ed.) (pp. 7-2–7-7). Chicago: Author.

Natural Resource Conservation Service. (2006a). *What is soil?* Retrieved July 19, 2007, from http://soils.usda.gov/education/facts/soil.html

Natural Resource Conservation Service. (2006b). *Soil formation and classification*. Retrieved July 19, 2007, from http://soils.usda.gov/education/facts/formation.htm

Reynolds, G. (2007, July). Produce sector urged to adopt supply chain coding standard. *Food Production Daily*. Retrieved July 23, 2007, from http://www.foodproductiondaily.com/news/ng.asp?id=74008

CHAPTER 4

FOOD SAFETY REGULATIONS AND PROGRAMS

Bonnie L. Gerald, PhD, DTR

Chapter Objectives

After reading the chapter and reflecting on the contents, you should be able to:

1. Understand the role of good manufacturing processes (GMPs), good hygiene practices (GHPs), and hazard analysis critical control point (HACCP) in achieving food safety objectives.
2. Describe the role of food safety controls in risk analysis.
3. Discuss the role of government agencies in assuring a safe food supply.
4. Describe the relationship between international and US food safety regulations.

Key Terms

GHP (good hygiene practices): A requirement for manufacturers of foods to assure that food products are safely handled.

GMP (good manufacturing processes): A requirement for manufacturers of foods (and medications) to assure that products are safely made.

HACCP (hazard analysis critical control point): A systematic preventive approach to food safety that addresses danger areas and serves as a means of prevention rather than finished product inspection.

Introduction

Globalization of the food supply has increased the movement of food across international boundaries. Commodities such as wheat can be shipped from midwestern states to Europe where they are processed into foods that are imported into the United States. A typical grocery store in the United States might have grapes from Chile, beef from Australia, shrimp from Indonesia, and pasta from Italy on its shelves. The United States receives about 25,000 shipments of imported food every day (Economic Research Service, 2006). Free trade has been beneficial to food producers worldwide; however, the flow of goods across international boundaries has created challenges for ensuring a safe food supply. Several factors determine the safety of food products: restricted shelf life, seasonality, consumer awareness, heterogeneity of food products, supply chain complexity, and low added value (Van der Spiegel, Luning, Ziggers, & Jongen, 2004).

> **Learning Point:** In 1987 a typical grocery store carried 173 produce items. In 2006 the typical grocery store carried about 345 produce items. (Economic Research Service, USDA; "Food Sector.")

Most food that is produced for domestic consumption is shipped across state lines. As the "food miles" increase, the potential for unsafe food also increases. The federal government has primacy over any state laws concerning food. Federal jurisdiction began in 1906 to 1907 with the passage of the Pure Food and Drug Act and the Federal Meat Inspection Act, respectively (*Harvard Law Review*, 2007). However, states are responsible for implementing federal guidelines. Fifteen federal agencies that are involved with food safety include the US Department of Agriculture (USDA); Department of Commerce, Food and Drug Administration (FDA); and Environmental Protection Agency (EPA). International organizations with food safety guidelines include the Codex Alimentarius Commission, the World Trade Organization, and the World Health Organization. This chapter will describe food safety regulations and policies of the major federal and international organizations. Current surveillance and inspection methods also will be discussed in the context of the US regulatory environment.

Traditional Inspection and Recalls

Several agencies are responsible for the safety of the US food supply. The USDA and the US Department of Health and Human Services (HHS) are cabinet-level government bodies with broad oversight of human food safety. Within the USDA is the Food Safety and Inspection Service (FSIS), which inspects all red meats, poultry, and eggs. The FDA, part of HHS, regulates all other foods. Marine fish and shellfish production is regulated by the Office of Seafood, which is housed within the FDA. Other agencies indirectly involved with assuring a safe food supply are the EPA and the Centers for Disease Control and Prevention (CDC).

> **Learning Point:** The Food and Drug Administration was formerly known as the Bureau of Chemistry.

Foods are inspected for wholesomeness. Traditional inspections occur at or near the endpoint of the food in the processing channel. The approach has been reactive, meaning that food is accepted or rejected as fit for human consumption upon inspecting the food. Proactive measures to limit hazards are a recent development in food safety procedures.

The current US food safety system has been criticized for overlapping regulations between agencies and inspection disparities between foods. For example, a meat processing plant is inspected daily, while a food processor making bakery items containing cheese is inspected every 6 months. Fruit and vegetables, which have been linked to *E. coli* outbreaks, are processed in plants that are only inspected twice per year.

The federal agency risk-based approach still considers meat products as potentially more hazardous than fruits and vegetables. However, recent foodborne illness outbreaks indicate the greatest threat to public health is from seafood, followed by fruits, vegetables, and eggs. Meats and poultry rank fourth in reported foodborne illness outbreaks but receive more funding for inspections and research than the previous three categories (US GAO, 2004).

Recommendations have been made to consolidate all agencies into a single food safety agency (Hammonds, 2004). Critics argue that one federal food safety agency would be more effective than the current system. Another perspective is that the current system, while not efficient, would be too costly to replace and could make the food system vulnerable to bioterrorism attacks during the consolidation process. Some observers recommend that the agencies receive more funding and regulatory authority instead of bureaucratic reorganization (*Harvard Law Review*, 2007). The National Uniformity for Food Act of 2005 addresses concerns about agency coordination for ensuring a safe food supply. The purpose of the legislation is to provide uniform warning notification requirements for food. It amends the Federal Food, Drug, and Cosmetic Act (FFDCA) to prevent states from promulgating food safety requirements that are not identical to FFDCA requirements. States can petition the federal government for an exemption to a uniformity requirement for situations unique to a specific area (H.R., 2006).

Recalls

FSIS conducts tests of meat, poultry, and egg products after they leave the slaughterhouse or processing plant and enter the food supply chain. Despite protection measures, an unsafe food can appear at the end of the supply chain. Food recalls are a collaboration between FSIS and the manufacturer. Foods are recalled voluntarily when it is determined by the government or by independent sources that a food can result in negative health consequences for consumers. A recall is a risk management tool that is used to protect consumers from potential harm from unsafe foods (FSIS, 2000). Foods can be recalled by the manufacturer if there is evidence of contamination ("adulteration") or if the food product does not match its label description ("misbranding"). Food recalls are voluntary. Neither the USDA nor the FDA has regulatory authority to require a company to recall its products (US GAO, 2004). Food manufacturers generally pull their products from shelves to protect their customers and to avoid negative publicity. FSIS works with manufacturers during the recall process to ensure that all products are removed from the food supply.

Food manufacturers conduct effectiveness checks during the recall to confirm that all outlets have removed the product according to the manufacturer's instructions. FSIS monitors the process to verify that adequate notice has been given and the manufacturer has taken reasonable measures to remove the recalled product (FSIS,

2004). An effective recall is one that recovers a large proportion of the product in a timely manner. Effectiveness measures used for evaluating the recall are recovery rate, completion time, and recovery rate–completion time ratio. A study of effectiveness indicators from 1994 to 2002 meat and poultry recalls showed no significant differences based on the size of manufacturing plant or type of meat processed. HACCP implementation facilitated recalls but did not appear to improve the effectiveness of the recalls (Hooker, Tertanavat, & Salin, 2005).

The federal government has developed a three-part risk analysis approach to the food supply: risk assessment, hazard identification, and assessment; risk management and pathogen reduction (PR)/ HACCP; and risk communication and protection tools for consumers and the supply chain (US GAO, 2000). FSIS has the responsibility for domestic and imported meat, poultry, and egg product recalls, while the FDA has responsibility for all other food product recalls. Tertanavat and Hooker (2004) examined the FSIS database of meat and poultry recalls for the period 1994 to 2002. They found that processed or cooked food accounted for 74% of all recalls. Beef was the most frequently recalled meat. The most common pathogens associated with recalled products were *Campylobacter jejuni/coli, E.coli* H157:07, *Salmonella,* and *Listeria monocytogenes.* The number of recalls and the amount of recalled product have been increasing since 1997, which might result from improved communication and monitoring by FSIS (Tertanavat & Hooker, 2004). Recalls are a risk management tool used in risk analysis. Risk analysis is part of US food safety controls.

Food Safety Controls

Public health has become the responsibility of governments worldwide. The United Nations' Food and Agriculture Organization (FAO) and the World Health Organization (WHO), working with the Codex Alimentarius Commission, developed the risk analysis framework as a means to establish food safety controls at the national level. Food safety controls are linked to the manufacturer and the consumer through the federal government's process of risk analysis. The food safety controls are national goals meant to provide guidance for policy making and for the private sector (Gorris, 2005). Federal agencies determine an *appropriate level of protection* (ALOP) for its citizens. The ALOP will guide formation of a *food safety objective* (FSO), which determines the allowable level of hazard that can be in a product up to the point of consumption (Gorris, 2005).

The incentive for developing FSOs is to make food safety practices transparent and quantifiable (Zwietering, 2005). Manufacturers can develop their own *performance objective* (PO), which is similar to the government's FSO. The measures are the link between manufacturers and the public (Gorris, 2005). Food safety management systems, such as HACCP, good hygiene practices (GHP), and good manufacturing processes (GMP), are tactics to meet the FSO. The effectiveness of food safety controls within and between nations is evaluated periodically at meetings of the Codex Committee on Food Hygiene (CCFH) of the Codex Alimentarius Commission (Codex), an international food safety organization. The United States is represented by delegates from the FDA. FSIS seeks public comment prior to the CCFH session through electronic dialog and face-to-face meetings in Washington, DC (FSIS, Federal Register, 2007). International health regulations are a legal framework to prevent or contain serious risks to public health. The regulations were developed by WHO to improve the global database for reported illness from biological, chemical, and radiological agents. The US Department of Health and Human Services has the primary responsibility for reporting US information to the WHO. The regulations can be modified based on sound science and technology (US HHS, 2007).

Food Safety Management Systems

FSOs help determine allowable limits or concentrations of a food hazard. Managing these limits through food safety management systems communicates to the public that risk is a continuum and cannot be reduced to zero. HACCP, GHP, and GMP are well-recognized tactics that were developed to meet FSOs. GHPs and GMPs must be implemented prior to using HACCP in food production.

GMPs were developed in the 1960s as part of the quality assurance (QA) trend. The purpose of GMPs is to ensure product consistency and quality that is appropriate for the product's intended use. The practices can be a general set of guidelines or specific procedures applied to either a vertical or horizontal food supply chain. The expected outcome is safe and hygienic food products (Institute of Food Science and Technology, 1991).

> **Learning Point:** Vertical integration refers to all elements of a supply chain controlled by one organization. Horizontal integration refers to products moving through a series of organizations that interact with each other.

GHPs were developed to facilitate sanitation and safety practices as foods move through the supply chain. The Codex Code of Hygienic Practice applies to produce, seafood, milk, and eggs. The guidance covers topics such as water reuse in processing plants, use of manure, and worker sanitation. The GHPs are revised periodically by Codex member nations based on most recent food safety research (Codex Alimentarius, 2006). HACCP is an example of a risk-based GHP.

HACCP was developed for NASA (National Aeronautics and Space Administration) to decrease the risk of astronauts becoming ill during a space flight. The food safety management system is endorsed by the National Academy of Sciences, the Codex Alimentarius Commission,

---

The seven HACCP principles are:

1. Analyze hazards—Potential hazards and methods to control the hazard.
2. Identify critical control points—Points in the food supply chain where a hazard can be controlled or eliminated.
3. Establish preventive measures with critical limits for each control point—Determine appropriate time and temperatures for safe food preparation.
4. Establish procedures to monitor the critical control points—How to measure and who will measure.
5. Establish corrective actions to be taken when monitoring shows that a critical limit has not been met—Appropriate safe actions such as discarding or reheating food.
6. Establish procedures to verify that the system is working properly—Conduct periodic checks for all time and temperature measuring devices.
7. Establish effective record keeping to document the HACCP system—Record hazards, monitor safety requirements, and verify actions taken (FDA, 2001).

and the National Advisory Committee on Microbiological Criteria for Foods.

The FDA has issued regulations establishing HACCP as the food safety management system for several parts of the food supply chain. Currently meat and poultry plants, juice processors, and seafood processors must use HACCP as part of their operations. Imported seafood also must be processed using an acceptable HACCP system to enter the US food supply (CFSAN, 2005). Eventually all parts of the food system, including imported foods, will be required to implement an HACCP program. Segments of the food system, such as retail food operations, health care, and the low-acid canned food industry, have voluntarily adopted HACCP principles.

Learning Point: The Pillsbury Corporation developed the HACCP concept for NASA in the 1960s.

Import Regulations

Both the USDA and the FDA regulate imported foods. The USDA requires foreign meatpacking plants to comply with US standards before entering the country. Imported meat is allowed in only 10 US ports. Restricting ports of entry has allowed the USDA to allocate its inspectors efficiently. The FDA does not restrict port of entry or border crossings for imported foods. Approximately 1% of imported foods under FDA jurisdiction are inspected. The FDA only has authority to stop imported food at the border (Imports flood in fast, 2007).

Imported fruits and vegetables are inspected by both the FDA and the USDA. Pest control is the responsibility of the USDA. The FDA inspects for produce safety and hygiene. The federal agencies have implemented a risk-based system for fruit and vegetable commodities subject to phytosanitary measures. The measures are port of entry inspection, approved postharvest treatment, certification from a pest-free area, and certification that risks can be mitigated through commercial practices (Reynolds, 2007).

The Public Health Security and Bioterrorism Act of 2002 requires domestic and foreign facilities that manufacture, process, pack, or hold food for human or animal consumption in the United States to register with the FDA, effective December 12, 2003.

Owners, operators, or agents in charge of domestic or foreign facilities that manufacture/process, pack, or hold food for human or animal consumption in the United States are required to register the facility with the FDA. Domestic facilities are required to register whether or not food from the facility enters interstate commerce. Foreign facilities that manufacture/process, pack, or hold food also are required to register unless food from that facility undergoes further processing (including packaging) by another foreign facility before the food is exported to the United States. However, if the subsequent foreign facility performs only a minimal activity, such as putting on a label, both facilities are required to register (FDA, 2002).

Private Food Standards

Outbreaks of foodborne illness from spinach, lettuce, peanut butter, and ground beef are examples of limited government oversight of the food supply. The FDA is responsible for the safety of 80% of the food supply, yet it lacks the manpower and regulatory authority to remove hazardous products. This situation has made food processors aware of the need to take responsibility for their products' safety. Some companies have established a system to trace ingredients back to their original sources. Other companies regularly test

---

Examples of FDA-regulated foods under the Bioterrorism Act of 2002

- food and food additives for man or animals
- dietary supplements and dietary ingredients
- infant formula
- beverages (including alcoholic beverages and bottled water)
- fruits and vegetables
- fish and seafood
- dairy products and shell eggs
- raw agricultural commodities for use as food or components of food
- canned foods
- live food animals
- bakery goods, snack food, and candy

Table 4.1 Federal Agency Food Safety Responsibilities

US Department of Agriculture	US Department of Health and Human Services	Environmental Protection Agency	US Department of the Treasury	US Department of Commerce	Federal Trade Commission
Food Safety and Inspection Service (meat and poultry) Agricultural Marketing Service (eggs, dairy, produce, meat and poultry products) Federal Grain Inspection Service (grain, rice) Animal and Plant Health Inspection Service (protect from diseases and pests) Agricultural Research Service (food safety research)	Food and Drug Administration (all food except meat, poultry, and eggs) Centers for Disease Control (investigate foodborne disease)	Regulate pesticides and establish pesticide tolerance levels	Bureau of Alcohol, Tobacco, and Firearms (alcoholic beverage control) US Customs Service (examine/collect food for other agencies)	National Marine Fisheries Service (voluntary seafood inspection)	Regulate advertising of food products

Source: US General Accounting Office. (1990). *Food safety and quality: Who does what in the federal government* (GAO/RCED-91-19B, pp. 4–5).

products for contaminants and pathogens. For example, one company's organic spinach was contaminated with *E. coli*, resulting in 204 illnesses and three deaths in 2006. The company now tests for pathogens along its supply chain from seeds to irrigation water to processed salad greens. The added cost of testing is the company's risk management tool to decrease the probability of liability claims and negative publicity (Carey, 2007).

The private food safety and quality standards are not legally binding for suppliers; however, the standards set by food processors have virtually become mandatory for suppliers. The private standards are the processors' response to the regulatory environment as well as a means of competitive positioning in the marketplace. Consumer fears appear to have a stronger influence on food processors than does governmental regulations (Henson & Reardon, 2005).

The food industry does recognize the importance of regulations for the following reasons:

- increasing consumer confidence in the food supply
- ensuring a consistent approach to food safety throughout the food chain
- providing guidance on food safety issues
- ensuring that suppliers and consumers are also fulfilling their roles with regard to food safety (Motarjemi & Mortimore, 2005)

Implicit in these reasons is the cooperation of government, industry, and consumers for managing food safety risks.

Limited government resources for inspection and enforcement, coupled with the rise of private standards and consumer concerns, have generated interest in coregulation of food safety issues. Coregulation governance of food safety is the cooperation between public and private sectors of the food supply in the process of creating new rules. The process can result in agreements, conventions, and legislation. However, a key to successful coregulation is understanding the public and private motives behind the governance, including potential costs and benefits (Martinez, Fearne, Caswell, & Henson, 2006). The United Kingdom, Canada, and the United States practice limited forms of coregulation. Constraints on effectiveness of the governance include timing of consultation with industry, inadequate research by governments, and potentially biased information generated by industry. The enforcement of food safety standards and monitoring the food supply might be the most effective use of coregulation.

Chapter Summary

An increasing reliance on processed foods has placed a greater burden on US agencies that are responsible for ensuring a safe food supply. Federal agencies have limited regulatory authority and rely on industry cooperation and consumer vigilance. The federal government is best positioned to resolve regulatory gaps and make appropriate policy decisions based on their impact and practical application. Food processors can facilitate the implementation of both private and public governance by instilling a culture of food safety throughout the organization. Validation and maintenance of the HACCP system also is a primary responsibility of food processors. Consumers should be educated on the differences between concept and risk and understand that all food cannot be tested. All stakeholders have a *shared responsibility* in the production of safe food (Motarjemi & Mortimore, 2005).

> **Learning Point:** WHO coined the term "shared responsibility," meaning collaboration between all sectors including government, consumer organizations, and food processors to achieve a safe and wholesome food supply.

Issues to Debate

1. Have the class search for examples of coregulation in the United States. Discuss the impact of the public–private governance. If you were to perform a cost–benefit analysis, who is the primary beneficiary of the coregulation?
2. Discuss the reasons for the disparity in funding support between the USDA and the FDA. Considering recent data that produce and seafood cause more foodborne illness than meat, how should the FDA monitor food under its jurisdiction? Is it practical to adopt the USDA's model?

3. Should the USDA and FDA be given more regulatory authority? Is there a disadvantage to these agencies having increased regulatory power?
4. Trace the path of cheese or lettuce as it moves through the food system. Identify the federal agencies involved with the safety of the food at each stage of the system. Discuss areas where the process could be modified to make the food less likely to be recalled.
5. Outbreaks of foodborne illness have been traced to imported produce, such as raspberries from Guatemala. Is it appropriate to impose food safety standards of the developed nations on less developed countries? Who is responsible for the safety of imported foods: the government or the importer?
6. Is it possible to implement HACCP as the only food safety system instead of traditional inspections for meat and poultry? Discuss the implications if this were done.

References

Carey, J. (2007, May 21). How safe is the food supply? *Business Week.*
Center for Food Safety and Applied Nutrition (CFSAN). (2005, May 13). *FDA's evaluation of the seafood HACCP program for fiscal years 2002/2003.* Retrieved July 12, 2007, from http://www.cfsan.fda.gov/~comm/seaval3.html
Codex Alimentarius. (2006). *Codex code of hygienic practice.* Retrieved November 9, 2007, from http://www.codexalimentarius.net/download/standards/10200/cxp_053e.pdf
Economic Research Service, USDA. (2006). *Food sector.* Retrieved June 20, 2007, from http://www.ers.usda.gov/browse/FoodSector.html
FDA. (2001). *HACCP: A state-of-the-art approach for food safety. FDA backgrounder.* Retrieved July 12, 2007, from http://www.cfsan.fda.gov/~lrd/bhhaccp.html
FDA. (2002). *Public health security and bioterrorism preparedness and response act of 2002.* Retrieved November 11, 2007, from http://www.fda.gov/oc/bioterrorism/PL107-188.html
Food Safety and Inspection Service (FSIS). (2000). *Food recalls: Food safety focus.* Retrieved from http://www.fsis.usda.gov/OA/pubs/recallfocus.htm
Food Safety and Inspection Service (FSIS). (2004). *Effectiveness checks* (FSIS Directive 8080.1 Rev.4, Attachment 3). Retrieved from http://www.fsis.usda.gov/OPPDE/rdad/FSISDirectives/8080_1/8080.1Rev4_Attach3.pdf
Food Safety and Inspection Service (FSIS). (2007, September 26). *Codex Alimentarius Commission: Meeting of Codex Committee on food hygiene*

(Federal Register Vol. 72, No. 186). Retrieved October 22, 2007, from http://www.fsis.usda.gov/OPPDE/rdad/FRPubs/2007-0036.htm

Gorris, L. G. M. (2005). Food safety objective: An integral part of food chain management. *Food Control, 16*, 801–809.

Hammonds, T. M. (2004). It is time to designate a single food safety agency. *Food and Drug L. J.,* 427–428.

Harvard Law Review. (2007). Reforming the food safety system: What if consolidation isn't enough? *120*(5), 1345–1366.

Henson, S., & Reardon, T. (2005). Private agri-food standards: Implications for food policy and the agri-food system. *Food Policy, 30*, 241–253.

Hooker, N. H., Tertanavat, R. P., & Salin, V. (2005). Crisis management effectiveness indicators for US meat and poultry recalls. *Food Policy, 30*, 63–80.

House of Representatives (H.R.). (2006, February 28). *National uniformity of food act of 2005* (Report 109-379 109th Congress, 2nd session).

Imports flood in fast, but the agency lacks funds, authority. (2007, May 4). *USA Today.*

Institute of Food Science and Technology. (1991). *Food and drink: Good manufacturing practice: A guide to its responsible management.* London: IFST.

Martinez, M. G., Fearne, A., Caswell, J. A., & Henson, S. (2006). Co-regulation as a possible model for food safety governance: Opportunities for public–private partnerships. *Food Policy, 32*(3), 299–314.

Mortarjemi, Y., & Mortimore, S. (2005). Industry's need and expectations to meet food safety, 5th international meeting: Noordwijk food safety and HACCP forum 9–10 December 2002. *Food Control, 16*, 523–529.

Reynolds, G. (2007, July 17). Risk-based inspections for commodity imports announced. *FoodUSA Food Production Daily.* Retrieved July 23, 2007, from http://www.foodproductiondaily-usa.com/news/printNewsBis .asp?id=78268

Tertanavat, R., & Hooker, R. H. (2004). Understanding the characteristics of US meat and poultry recalls: 1994–2002. *Food Control, 15*, 359–367.

US Department of Health and Human Services. (2007). *Revised international health regulations are effective for US.* Retrieved November 10, 2007, from http://www.globalhealth.gov/ihr

US General Accounting Office (GAO). (2000). *Food safety. Actions needed by USDA and FDA to ensure that companies promptly carry out recalls* (GAO/RCED-00-195).

US General Accounting Office (GAO). (2004). *Federal food safety and security system: Fundamental restructuring is needed to address fragmentation and overlap* (GAO-04-588T, p. 18).

Van der Spiegel, M., Luning, P. A., Ziggers, G. W., & Jongen, W. M. F. (2004). Evaluation of performance measurement instruments on their use for food quality systems. *Critical Reviews in Food Science and Nutrition, 44*, 501–512.

Zwietering, M. (2005). Practical considerations on food safety objectives. *Food Control, 16*, 818–823.

CHAPTER 5

FUTURE FOOD SAFETY INITIATIVES AND BIOTECHNOLOGY

Bonnie L. Gerald, PhD, DTR

Chapter Objectives

After reading the chapter and reflecting on the contents, you should be able to:

1. Describe the role of transparency in the food supply chain.
2. Understand benefits and limitations of technology applied to food safety issues.
3. Describe food safety initiatives from a global perspective.

Key Terms

biotechnology: New finds in science related to agriculture, food science, and medicine.

food packaging: Supplies, such as plastic and aluminum containers, Styrofoam, and other wrapping.

food supply chain: A worldwide network of food producers, processors, and distributors.

food systems: Includes everything from farm to table.

international regulations: Governmental bodies that are developing regulations to improve food safety and consistency throughout the global community.

Introduction

The US food system will continue to experience challenges of safety and integrity. Contributing factors are the increasing complexity of the food supply chain, prevalence of manufactured food products, increased food imports, and intensive agricultural production (Van der Spiegel, Luning, Ziggers, & Jongen, 2004). Acceptable levels of food safety risk also are influenced by consumer expectations of quality, shelf life, security, and price. Packaging technology has improved the safety of some foods while introducing potential risks to other foods. The potential for deliberate contamination has stimulated a variety of food defense initiatives. This chapter will assess recent biological and technical food safety measures and their potential impact on the food system. The influence of international food safety regulations also will be evaluated in the context of recent innovations in food safety.

Farm-to-Fork System

The farm-to-fork perspective of food safety encompasses all aspects of food production and distribution. Farm to fork includes the key stages of harvesting, storage, processing, packaging, sales, and consumption (Domenech, Escriche, & Martorell, 2007). These key stages can be further defined as unit operations (Figure 5.1). Food can become unsafe at any stage in the food supply chain. At the farm end of the food supply chain, interventions using good agricultural practices (GAPs), such as clean water and animal vaccines, have reduced incidents of bacterial contamination. However, GAPs cannot reduce pathogens to insignificant levels (Sperber, 2005). It is at the processed product stage, in the middle of the supply chain, that the safety of the food is most likely to be compromised. The processing stage also presents opportunities to control hazards, the stage HACCP was first applied. Processors typically collect food ingredients from more than one source. Even a small amount of contaminated food can spread pathogens through an entire batch or throughout the plant. If good manufacturing practices (GMPs) are not used during processing, HACCP systems alone will not ensure safe food. Examples of GMPs include facility design, employee training, preventative maintenance, cleaning, and supplier approval. Opportunities to control hazards through processes such as cooking, drying, acidification, or refining occur at the processing stage. HACCP, when combined with GAPs and GMPs, should be the

Learning Point: Farm-to-fork food safety can include all of these steps (Buelens, Broens, Folstar, & Hofstede, 2005):

- raw material intake
- sorting and grading
- trimming and cutting
- slaughter
- packing
- cooling/chilling or freezing
- physical–chemical processes
- drying/conditioning
- milling/crushing/extraction
- sprouting
- washing/decontamination
- microbiological processes
- packing
- storage and transport
- waste disposal

FIGURE 5.1 Farm to Fork

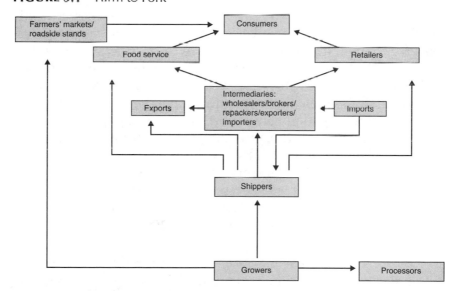

Source: Available at: www.ers.usda.gov/publications/aer830/aer830.pdf. Retrieved on 1/2/08.

context of food safety measures in the farm-to-fork system (Sperber, 2005; Burlingame & Pineiro, 2007).

Transparency

At the consumption end of the food chain, consumers expect quality products. Food quality can be defined as "fitness for consumption." The food processors' interpretation of food quality includes nutrition, sensory characteristics, and marketing attributes. Consumers perceive food quality as the assumption of safety (absence of risk), conformity to product definition (not mislabeled or adulterated), and produced ethically (animal welfare or workers' rights) in addition to the processor definitions (Peri, 2005). The public assumes that food safety measures are applied at each stage in the supply chain, but given the frequency of reported incidents of food contamination, how can we be sure they are, and by whom?

Food chain suppliers have responded to consumer demand and governmental oversight by implementing transparency measures in their systems. Transparency of a supply chain is the extent all stakeholders have in a shared understanding and access to requested product and process information without loss, noise, delay, or distortion (Hofstede, 2002). To achieve transparency, businesses within the food supply chain establish organizational and technical systems for communication within and between businesses about their quality control and tracking systems. The use of molecular biology (DNA methods such as polymerase chain reaction [PCR]) for quality control analysis in conjunction with production and management data creates information networks within food supply chains (Beulens, Broens, Folstar, & Hofstede, 2005). The information generated must share identification standards within the supply chain network as well as comply with government regulations. For example, the PCR method has been used successfully to detect *Listeria monocytogenes* in salmon. The PCR method can generate results within 24–48 hours (Becker, Jordan, & Holzapfel, 2005).

> **Learning Point:** Polymerase chain reaction (PCR) is a laboratory detection method using DNA.

Barriers to transparency include unauthorized use of information, uncertainty about cost savings, and loss of independence. The issues of functionality, transparency, and connectivity must be addressed when establishing food safety monitoring and tracking systems within the food supply chain.

Traceability is an essential part of transparency. The ability of the food industry to trace and follow feed, food, and food-producing animals through all stages of production, processing, and distribution is an outcome of consumer demands for information and concerns about bioterrorism (Thompson, Sylvia, & Morrissey, 2005). Traceability in the United States is limited to voluntary product recall procedures and mandatory documentation. Increased Class I product recalls, considered to be high health risk cases, have doubled from 1993 to 2003. The increase suggests that current practices are inadequate. Establishing traceability guidelines could decrease the cost of foodborne illness. Implementing food supply chain traceability will require compatibility (ability to communicate), data standardization (establish measurement parameters within the chain), and an accepted traceable resource unit (TRU). A TRU is a unit of trade, such as one case of lettuce or one truckload of frozen fish (Thompson, Sylvia, & Morrissey, 2005). A recent TRU tracking method is radio frequency identification (RFID). The RFID tags do not require manual scanning, allowing hundreds of tags to be downloaded at one time. Information such as temperature readings and product movement within the supply chain can be stored on the tag (Thompson, Sylvia, & Morrissey, 2005).

Public and Private Initiatives

Governments and the public also have a role in the flow of information in the food supply chain. Recent advances in food safety research and expanded media coverage have increased consumer awareness of potential hazards. The increasing purchase of processed foods, expanding international trade, and growing awareness of food safety hazards have fueled incentives for public intervention in the food supply chain (Lipton, Sinha, & Blackmon, 2002). The public and private sectors have created partnerships to address food safety issues. The US meat industry worked with the USDA to develop HACCP plans for small processors. The financial burden of developing HACCP plans on their own could have resulted in closures of small meat processors. The private sector also uses third-party certification of hazard management as part of procurement. The specification of food safety standards is becoming prevalent within the US food supply as well as a condition for international trade. The public sector can provide training, production guidelines (instead of mandated standards), and certification services (Unnevehr & Roberts, 2002). For example, the government of Bangladesh provided assistance to its seafood industry so that it could meet international food safety standards (Cato & Dos Santos, 2000).

Consumer perception of risks differs from those of experts. Experts might perceive a risk as scientifically negligible as a result of toxicological analysis. Consumers view media reports of contamination, regardless of concentration or effect, as equally risky. Experts' dismissal of "negligible risk" does little to inspire consumer confidence in scientists and governmental agencies (Anklam & Battaglia, 2001). The "perception filter" of subjectivity acts as a mirror that reflects, deflects, or distorts factual information. A food safety risk might be perceived as involuntary (unknowingly contaminated), catastrophic (affecting many people simultaneously), or unnatural (technical). These psychological factors will influence consumer reaction to hazards (Verbeke, Frewer, Scholderer, & De Brabander, 2007). The public and private sectors use several approaches to counteract these perceptions.

Mandatory labeling and traceability measures, while helpful in the event of a food safety incident, have not generated much public interest. However, quality labels or safety guarantees on a product seem to be more highly valued because they facilitate decision making, including the decision to avoid a product. Generic food safety information is likely to be ignored by consumers because they cannot see it fulfilling a personal need. Delivering safety information of a perceived high relevance to specific segments of the population might be effective in changing consumer behavior. However, this approach will require further identification of consumer segments. Consumer participation via focus groups, public hearings, and conferences is a tool for policy making when a potential exists for environmental or human exposure to hazards (Verbeke et al., 2007). Proactive communication about emerging food safety issues might increase consumer confidence in risk management practices (Van Kleef et al., 2006).

Primary Packaging Initiatives

Packaging is a widely used method of protecting both minimally and highly processed foods. Its primary functions are for protection and extended shelf life. The packaging can serve as a barrier, a scavenger, or as a system capable of responding to changing conditions. Several levels of packaging are used by processors.

Learning Point: Packaging types include:

- Primary—direct food contact, such as cans, bottles, and plastic bags
- Secondary—encase primary packaging, such as cardboard boxes
- Tertiary—bundle secondary into larger containers or use of overwrap. This form is used for protection during transport and storage.

Primary packaging is especially relevant to food safety. FDA approval is required for all packaging materials that have direct food contact. There can be no migration of packaging material to the food. Examples of migration include laminates sticking to food and bottled water contaminated by plastic molecules from the bottle. Packaging can be active or passive. See Table 5.1 for more information on packaging materials.

Packaging—Passive

Passive packaging includes vacuum, modified atmosphere packaging, and controlled atmosphere packaging. Food packed under vacuum has all oxygen removed within the package. The food can be stored at 40°F for no more than 10 days. Low-acid foods or foods that support growth of botulinum toxin (anaerobes) cannot use this type of packaging. Sous-vide is a form of vacuum packaging. Modified atmosphere packaging (MAP) is widely used for minimally processed fresh produce. The modified gas atmosphere within the package combined with refrigerated storage temperatures extends the product's shelf life. The CO_2 produced by respiration lowers the

Table 5.1   Primary Packaging

Packaging	Technology or function
Glass	Made from silicon dioxide. Container tops are hermetically sealed by metal caps.
Metal	Steel or aluminum is hermetically sealed.
Paper	Bags laminated for burst (wet) strength prevent moisture loss, and are grease and tear resistant. Paperboard lined with plastic (milk cartons). Waxed fiberboard (fresh poultry or produce).
Plastic	Polyethylene—Flexible, barrier to light and moisture (plastic bags). Polypropylene—Inside layer of packages subject to high temperatures (retort pouches). Polystyrene—Cushioning, insulation (egg cartons, cups, and plates). Polyvinylchloride—Heat resistance (prevents spattering from microwavable containers).
Other	Edible films—Part of food (sausage casing); thin polysaccharide or protein layer (dried fruits). Laminates—Multiple layers of foil, paper, or plastic acting as barriers to oxygen, water, and light (sauces, snack foods). Foil—Vapor and moisture barrier (aseptic packaging).

product's pH, which generally has an antimicrobial effect. There have been concerns regarding growth of facultatively anaerobic bacteria within MAP, particularly *Listeria monocytogenes*. Studies indicate that MAP vegetables such as lettuce and cabbage can support multiple *L. monocytogenes* serotypes with different levels of resistance to acid and heat (Francis & O'Beirne, 2005). Controlled atmosphere packaging allows oxygen and carbon dioxide exchange within the package. Fresh produce can be packaged using controlled atmosphere technology. Sachets or pads within the container have been a successful application of passive technology. Three forms are used: oxygen absorbers, moisture absorbers, and ethanol vapor generators. The sachets/pads have been used in pasta, bakery, produce, and meat packaging (Appendini & Hotchkiss, 2002).

Packaging—Active

Consumers want preservative-free, long shelf life foods. Active packaging is a result of consumer demands for fresh, minimally processed, and safe food. The technology responds to changes in the package environment. This type of packaging controls produce maturation and ripening, helps achieve color development in meats, and extends shelf life. An active system using a desiccant will begin absorbing moisture when the relative humidity reaches a specified level within a package (Packaging gets active, 2004). Other examples of active technology include edible barriers to prevent browning in cut fresh fruits and vegetables, oxygen/carbon dioxide scavenging, microwave susceptor films (allow browning, crispness), steam release films, and time–temperature indicators to detect safety hazards.

Oxygen scavengers are now incorporated into the food label or directly into the package structure. Films for MAP of meat have oxygen scavengers within the film. Oxidizable resins such as ethylene methyl acrylate cyclohexane methyl acrylate (EMCM) use ultraviolet (UV) light to remove excess oxygen. Polyethylene terephthalate PET plastics are replacing glass packaging. The PET also uses oxygen scavengers within the container wall.

Antimicrobial additives in packaging are used to slow microbial growth in foods. The FDA regulates use of antimicrobial additives incorporated into food packaging. One of the most effective antimicrobial additives is silver-substituted zeolite. The sodium ions in zeolite are substituted by silver ions. Zeolites are incorporated into polyethylene, polypropylene, and nylon (Appendini & Hotchkiss, 2002). Silver-based antimicrobial additives are activated at the package surface by moisture. The microbes exchange ions with the silver, thus limiting microbial growth. Other antimicrobial additives approved by the FDA for incorporation into package material are ethyl alcohol and chlorine dioxide. These materials volatilize throughout the package interior, which might be more effective than products activated by surface contact.

Another packaging material option for processors is an engineered polymer that is capable of absorbing or releasing moisture, oxygen, or antimicrobial agents to the food by means of microscopic channels within the polymer. The polymer is available as a film, a container, or a molded part (Packaging gets active, 2004). Future developments will hinge on the availability of new polymer materials, antimicrobials, appropriate testing methods, and government regulation. Developing coatings/binders that are compatible with polymers, combined with encapsulation, will be the focus of future research. An ideal future "smart" package would sense microbes and release controlled amounts of antimicrobial agents that have a wide range of activity and low toxicity. However, antimicrobial packaging should be considered part of hurdle technology, which includes more traditional methods of food processing controls, not a substitute for GMPs (Appendini & Hotchkiss, 2002).

Other Food Safety Processing Methods

Food safety applications for edible coatings are a result of technical advances in food processing. Heat and irradiation are two methods of maintaining product safety that have been used for many years by food processors. Although they are effective in controlling microbial growth, heat processing and irradiation have resulted in undesirable side effects such as taste and texture changes. Several new techniques have been developed that control pathogen growth yet maintain the desired sensory properties of the food.

Edible Coatings

Fresh produce respires until it is cooked for consumption, processed for preservation, or consumed fresh. The presence of moisture, oxygen, and carbon dioxide is a factor that determines the shelf life of harvested fruits and vegetables. Edible coatings, such as waxes and oils, have long been used to control moisture loss. Produce is sprayed or dipped in a coating mixture to produce a semipermeable membrane on the surface of the food. More recent applications are the addition of functional ingredients such as nutraceuticals and antimicrobials to coating formulations.

Polysaccharide and protein-based coatings have shown potential as antimicrobial carriers. Carageenan, a polysaccharide extracted from seaweed, has acted as a carrier for food-grade microbials such as lysozyme, nisin, grape seed extract, and EDTA. The carageenan–antimicrobial combination has been shown to reduce microorganism levels on fresh cut apples. Chitosan, a coating derived from shell materials of crustaceans and insects, contains the antifungal enzyme chitinase. The coating has successfully controlled pathogens on strawberries and raspberries. Zein, a corn protein, forms a shellac-like coating on nuts, dried fruit, and fresh produce. It acts as a barrier to microorganisms such as *Listeria monocytogenes*. Common antimicrobial agents used by food processors, such as benzoic acid, sodium benzoate, sorbic acid, potassium sorbate, and propionic acid, have been incorporated into coatings. Future coating formulations will contain the best properties of several materials, such as a patented combination of protein, glycerol, and organic acids to maintain quality and safety. The patented coating has demonstrated the ability to inhibit growth of *L. monocytogenes, S. gaminara,* and *E. coli* O157:H7 (Lin & Zhao, 2007). The use of edible coatings with antimicrobial properties is not widespread among processors. This might be due to factors such as compromised moisture barrier function of the coating, the primary purpose of edible coatings. More research is needed to develop coatings with stable adhesion and durability properties.

Thermal Processing

Two premises are the basis of thermal processing: (1) the heat resistance of microorganisms for a specific product, and (2) the heating rate of the specific product (Awuah, Ramaswamy, & Economides, 2007). Infrared heating has long been used by food processors to dry cereal products and thick foods such as potatoes. Using infrared heat to surface pasteurize meat products was shown to be effective in destroying *L. monocytogenes* without affecting the meat's color. The process could be used to control *L. monocytogenes* prior to final packaging of ready-to-eat meat and poultry products (Huang, 2004). Retort pouches are used for an increasing variety of foods in response to consumer demands for convenience. However, conventional thermal processing can negatively affect the food's sensory properties. Variable retort temperatures (VRTs) show promise to improve quality while controlling microbial growth. More testing and computer modeling are needed to determine optimal processing times for the nonuniform shape of retort pouches (Auwah, Ramaswamy, & Economides, 2007).

Irradiation

The technology for irradiation of food has existed since the 1930s. Research conducted in the 1950s by the Atomic Energy Commission (now the Department of Energy) determined the most effective use of irradiation was control of pathogenic microorganisms on food. The FDA considers irradiation to be a food additive and regulates the process as such. Any irradiated food must be labeled as "treated by irradiation" or "treated by ionizing energy" in addition to having the radura, the international symbol for irradiation, on the package. The FDA has approved irradiation for red meat, poultry, shell eggs, dried spices, wheat flour, and fresh produce. Irradiation is the application of ionizing energy (photons) to foods. Harmful microorganisms are destroyed without heating the food within the packaging. "Cold pasteurization" is another term used for irradiation.

Learning Point: Irradiation was studied for potential applications as part of President Eisenhower's "Atoms for Peace" program in the 1950s. Flour was the first food approved for irradiation by the FDA in 1963. Gamma rays can be generated from either an e-beam electron accelerator or radioactive isotopes (cobalt or cesium). However, foods cannot become radioactive as a result of irradiation. The amount of energy generated from photons to treat food is too low to cause the food to become radioactive.

Bacteria are destroyed by direct photon disruption of their DNA and by creation of free radicals, which damage their cell structure. The free radicals generated by irradiation can affect food quality by creating off-flavors and odors, reducing the gelling capacity of starches, and causing loss of vitamins A, C, E, and B1 when oxygen is present (Murano, 2003). Irradiation also might cause undesirable changes to polymer packaging materials. Plastic molecules can migrate from the package to the food, or the package integrity might be compromised as an outcome of irradiation. It appears that polymer reactions to irradiation are highly variable, dependent on specific combinations of product and packaging. Nuclear magnetic resonance (NMR) spectroscopy has shown polystyrene to be the most resistant of current packaging materials to irradiation (Pentimalli et al., 2000). The technology has not been widely adopted by food processors due to concerns about consumer acceptance of irradiated foods and the economics of large-scale use.

Nanotechnology

Nanotechnology is the study of manipulation of materials at the atomic, molecular, and macromolecular scale. The greater surface area compared to molecules with the same chemistry makes nanoparticles more biologically active. Nanotechnology has many potential applications from consumer electronics to nutraceuticals. Food processors could use nanosensors in foods to detect contamination or nanoparticles to deliver antimicrobials. However, information is limited on the risks of handling and consuming materials of ultrasmall scale. An assessment of safety and health risks so appropriate regulations can be developed is needed before nanotechnology use is widespread in the food supply chain (Chau, Wu, & Yen, 2007).

Biotechnology

Food biotechnology has the potential to create safer food; however, the process has generated controversy in the United States and Europe. It is the technology of manipulating DNA for the purpose of improving the quality and/or safety of foods (Murano, 2003). Bacteria typically are used in the process because they have no nuclei. The FDA regulates biotechnology-derived foods except red meat, poultry, and eggs, which are regulated by the USDA. Mandatory labeling for genetically modified foods is required if the food is changed significantly from its conventional counterpart. Examples of significantly modified foods are changes in nutritional composition or introduction of potential allergens. Genetically modified corn, soybeans, potatoes, canola, and papaya are grown in the United States.

One of the early FDA-approved genetically modified foods was the FLAVR SAVR tomato, which was modified to prolong shelf life. Biotechnology also is used to suppress toxic compounds produced by some plants. For example, cyanogenic compounds in cassava can cause chronic illness if not cooked properly. Cassava is a staple food in parts of Africa, thus it is important for maintaining the nutritional status of significant populations. A variety of cassava with lower levels of the toxic compound were produced through genetic engineering.

Beyond control of spoilage and reducing toxic compounds in foods, biotechnology has the potential to reduce harmful microorganisms on food. Several applications of biotechnology are being evaluated for their potential impact on food safety. Probiotics are a strain of bacteria living in the gut of animals, which can aid in digestion of feed. Probiotic bacteria that is genetically engineered to produce substances that inhibit growth of pathogens in an animal's intestinal tract could reduce incidents of contaminated meat and dairy products. Starter bacterial cultures used for producing fermented dairy products, such as yogurt and buttermilk, also have pathogen-inhibiting properties. Genetically engineered lactobacilli produce quantities of nisin, an antimicrobial that is effective in controlling *Listeria monocytogenes*. DNA produced by genetic engineering can be used by quality assurance personnel to test for pathogens in food. A DNA probe analysis used engineered DNA sequences to test for a genetic match with a suspected microorganism (Murano, 2003).

More than 10 years after the first use of biotechnology and despite evidence of potential benefits, public scrutiny of genetically modified foods continues in the United States and Europe. Current FDA policy advises, but does not require, that genetically modified food producers should test their crops for toxicity, allergenicity, and nutritional variations. The European Union countries want mandatory labeling, health testing, and ecological testing of genetically modified foods. US trade representatives state that the safety record of US crops and the endorsements from science-based organizations are sufficient proof that genetically modified foods are safe, and testing should not be mandated. Cultural differences and Europe's experience with mad cow disease are two reasons for the disagreement over biotechnology (Krimsky & Murphy, 2002). See Table 5.2 for more information.

National and International Food Safety Initiatives

The prominence of food safety controls in public policy debate is based on both science and economic issues. Costs of food safety regulations include production costs, compliance costs, administrative costs paid by taxes, and opportunity costs from taxation (Antle, 1999). Of the estimated 76 million cases of foodborne illness reported annually in the United States, only 18% can be linked to known causes. Despite research and surveillance programs, much is

Table 5.2 Genetically Modified Food Products: Benefits and Controversies

Benefits	Controversies
Crops	**Safety**
Enhanced taste and quality	Potential human health impact: allergens, transfer of antibiotic resistance markers, unknown effects
Reduced maturation time	
Increased nutrients, yields, and stress tolerance	Potential environmental impact: unintended transfer of transgenes through cross pollination, unknown effects on other organisms (e.g., soil microbes), and loss of flora and fauna biodiversity
Improved resistance to disease, pests, and herbicides	
New products and growing techniques	**Access and intellectual property**
	Domination of world food production by a few companies
Animals	Increasing dependence on industrialized nations by developing countries
Increased resistance, productivity, hardiness, and feed efficiency	Biopiracy—foreign exploitation of natural resources
Better yields of meat, eggs, and milk	**Ethics**
Improved animal health and diagnostic methods	Violation of natural organisms' intrinsic values
Environment	Tampering with nature by mixing genes among species
"Friendly" bioherbicides and bioinsecticides	Objections to consuming animal genes in plants and vice versa
Conservation of soil, water, and energy	Stress for animal
Bioprocessing for forestry products	**Labeling**
	Not mandatory in some countries (e.g., United States)
Better natural waste management	Mixing genetically modified crops with non-genetically modified crops confounds labeling attempts
More efficient processing	
Society	**Society**
Increased food security for growing populations	New advances might be skewed to interests of rich countries

Source: Retrieved January 2, 2008, from http://www.ornl.gov/sci/techresources/Human_Genome/elsi/gmfood.shtml.

unknown about how food becomes unsafe and causes foodborne illness. The 2007 Farm Bill has several provisions related to food safety. One creates a bipartisan Congressional Food Safety Commission to make recommendations for consistent regulations across agencies and determine the level of funding for federal agencies to fulfill their food safety mandates. Research funding was increased for biosecurity response planning and biotechnology risk assessment (McEntire & Davis, 2007).

The FDA is implementing a Food Protection Plan to identify potential hazards before harm can occur. The plan uses farm-to-fork risk analysis to prevent unintentional and deliberate contamination. The Food Protection Plan has three elements:

1. prevent foodborne contamination through risk identification and increased corporate responsibility
2. intervene at critical points in the food supply chain based on risk surveillance
3. respond rapidly to minimize harm through improved communication to all stakeholders (von Eschenbach, 2007)

An example of Food Protection Plan implementation is the National Antimicrobial Resistance Monitoring System (NARMS) for Enteric Bacteria. It is a collaboration between the CDC, the FDA, and the USDA to monitor changes in pathogens in animals and humans (Doyle, 2006).

It must be acknowledged, however, that even heavily regulated borders or ports of entry cannot assure complete protection from pathogens. A farm-to-fork situation awareness model has been proposed as a starting point for planning for widespread contamination of the US food supply. It would require sensors in the food processing stage that are capable of transmitting information to microprocessor voltage (the most common method of transmission), an integrated tracking system of all foods, and a software program capable of evaluating all food system information to determine probability of contamination. The concept is similar to war game scenarios or crisis simulation. It would require coordination between disparate public and private entities that is not technically feasible in the early 21st century (Lindberg, Grimes, & Giles, 2005).

The food supply chain is global. Growing international trade, higher standards in industrialized countries, and increased private sector responses will be important influences on the global food supply. Collaboration between the World Trade Organization, Codex Alimentarius Commission, economic organizations such as the European Union, and the private sector is needed to establish an effective, equitable, and sustainable food safety system (Stringer et al, 2007). The world's research, industry, and government sectors will have to respond to the challenges of:

- how well the food industry is responding to incentives for food safety improvement
- public intervention improving food market performance
- mitigation of food safety barriers so that global trade is facilitated (Unnevehr & Roberts, 2002)

Chapter Summary

The United States will continue to face challenges to the integrity of the food supply. Globalization of the food supply, promulgation of international regulations, and the rise of technology in food production will require the federal government to have the ability to respond quickly to the changing environment. Older technology such as plastic packaging and irradiation will be used in conjunction with cutting-edge methods such as nanotechnology and biotechnology to assure safety of the food supply. The federal government will form stronger collaborative relationships with international agencies whether a single food safety agency is created or the present system is retained.

Issues to Debate

1. Have the class search for opinions of biotechnology from scientists and consumer groups (both Europe and the United States). Divide the class into "pro" and "con" groups and have them present perspectives from both sides. At the end of the information sharing, have students express their own opinions on biotechnology, particularly its effect on food safety.
2. The general consensus among nations is to have equivalent food safety standards to facilitate trade. However, developing countries might find this difficult to achieve. Do the developed

countries have an obligation to help poor countries improve their food safety practices? If so, what should be done?

3. Transparency and traceability seem to be reasonable goals for the US food supply chain. Have the class discuss the barriers to implementation. Would transparency negatively affect innovation? How could transparency affect investors (stock market)? Would transparency really make the food supply safer?

4. Nanotechnology has limited regulation to date. Have the class locate information on nanotechnology food applications. Based on what is known, how should food nanotechnology be regulated?

5. The European Union has a single food safety agency. In the United States, multiple federal and state agencies implement food safety guidelines and regulations, which sometimes contradict one another. Should the United States combine all food safety programs into one agency? Discuss the advantages and disadvantages of a single food safety agency, including the impact to international trade.

References

Anklam, E., & Battaglia, R. (2001). Food analysis and consumer protection. *Trends in Food Science & Technology, 12*, 197–202.

Antle, J. M. (1999). Benefits and costs of food safety regulation. *Food Policy, 24*, 605–623.

Appendini, P., & Hotchkiss, J. H. (2002). Review of antimicrobial food packaging. *Innovative Food Science & Emerging Technologies, 3*, 113–126.

Awuah, G. B., Ramaswamy, H. S., & Economides, A. (2007). Thermal processing and quality: Principles and overview. *Chemical Engineering and Processing, 46*, 584–602.

Becker, B., Jordan, S., & Holzapfel, W. H. (2005). Rapid and specific detection of *Listeria monocytogenes* in smoked salmon with BAX®-PCR. *Food Control, 16*, 717–721.

Buelens, A. J. M., Broens, D. F., Folstar, P., & Hofstede, G. J. (2005). Food safety and transparency in food chains and networks: Relationships and challenges. *Food Control, 16*, 481–486.

Burlingame, B., & Pineiro, M. (2007). The essential balance: Risks and benefits in food safety and quality. *Journal of Food Composition and Analysis, 20*, 139–146.

Cato, J. C., & Dos Santos, C. A. L. (2000). Costs to upgrade the Bangladesh frozen shrimp processing sector to adequate technical and sanitary standards. In L. J. Unnevehr (Ed.), *The economics of HACCP.* St. Paul, MN: Eagan Press.

Chau, C. F., Wu, S. H., & Yen, G. C. (2007). The development of regulations for food nanotechnology. *Trends in Food Science and Technology, 18*, 269–280.

Domenech, E., Escriche, I., & Martorell, S. (2007). Quantification of risks to consumers' health and to companies' incomes due to failures in food safety. *Food Control, 18*, 1419–1427.

Doyle, M. P. (2006). Dealing with antimicrobial resistance. *Food Technology, 60*, 22–29.

Francis, G. A., & O'Beirne, D. (2005). Variation among strains of *Listeria monocytogenes*: Differences in survival on packaged vegetables and in response to heat and acid conditions. *Food Control, 16*, 687–694.

Hofstede, G. J. (2002). Transparency in netchains. In E. van Amerongen et al. (Eds.), *The challenge of global chains, proceedings of symposium Mercurius* (pp. 73–89). Wageningen, The Netherlands: Wageningen Academic Publishers.

Huang, L. (2004). Infrared surface pasteurization of turkey frankfurters. *Innovative Food Science and Emerging Technologies, 5*, 345–351.

Krimsky, S., & Murphy, N. K. (2002). Biotechnology at the dinner table: FDA's oversight of transgenic food. *Annals of the American Academy of Political & Social Science, 584*, 80–96.

Lin, D., & Zhao, Y. (2007). Innovations in the development and application of coatings for fresh and minimally processed fruits and vegetables. *Comprehensive Reviews in Food Science and Food Safety, 6*, 60–75.

Lindberg, D. V., Grimes, C. A., & Giles, C. L. (2005). Farm-to-table: A situation model for food safety assurance for porous borders. *Comprehensive Reviews of Food Science and Food Safety, 4*, 31–33.

Lipton, M., Sinha, S., & Blackman, R. (2002). Reconnecting agricultural technology to human development. *Journal of Human Development, 3*(1), 123–152.

McEntire, J. C., & Davis, S. F. (2007). The 2007 Farm Bill and its impact on food science. *Food Technology*. Retrieved December 27, 2007, from www.ift.org

Murano, P. S. (2003). *Understanding food science and technology*. Belmont, CA: Wadsworth/Thompson Learning.

Packaging gets active: Additives lead the way. (2004). *Plastics, Additives, and Compounds, 6*, 22–25.

Pentimalli, M., Capitani, D., Ferrando, A., Ferri, D., Ragni, P., & Segre, A. L. (2000). Gamma irradiation of food packaging materials: An NMR study. *Polymer, 41*, 2871–2881.

Peri, C. (2005). The universe of food quality. *Food Quality and Preference, 17*, 3–8.

Sperber, W. H. (2005). HACCP does not work from farm to table. *Food Control, 16*, 511–514.

Stringer, M. F., Hall, M. N., Betts, R., Edwards, N., Hall, M., Hughes, C., et al. (2007). A generic model of the integrated food supply chain to aid the investigation of food safety breakdowns. *Food Control, 18*, 755–765.

Thompson, M., Sylvia, G., & Morrissey, M. T. (2005). Seafood traceability in the United States: Current trends, system design, and potential applications. *Comprehensive Reviews in Food Science and Food Safety, 1*, 1–7.

Unnevehr, L. J., & Roberts, T. (2002). Food safety incentives in a changing world food system. *Food Control, 13,* 73–76.

Van der Spiegel, M., Luning, P. A., Ziggers, G. W., & Jongen, W. M. (2004). Evaluation of performance measurement instruments on their use for food quality systems. *Critical Reviews in Food Science and Nutrition, 44,* 501–512.

Van Kleef, E., Frewer, L. J., Chryssochoidis, G. M., Houghton, J. R., Korzen-Bohr, S., Krystallis, T., et al. (2006). Perceptions of food risk management among key stakeholders: Results from a cross-European study. *Appetite, 47,* 46–63.

Verbeke, W., Frewer, L. J., Scholderer, J., & De Brabander, H. F. (2007). Why consumers behave as they do with respect to food safety and risk information. *Analytica Chemica Acta, 586,* 2–7.

von Eschenbach, A. C. (2007). FDA's new approach to food protection. *Food Technology.* Retrieved December 27, 2007, from www.ift.org

SECTION TWO

FOOD INSECURITY

CHAPTER 6

THE MEASUREMENT OF FOOD INSECURITY IN THE UNITED STATES

Craig Gundersen, PhD

Chapter Objectives

After reading the chapter and reflecting on the contents, you should be able to:

1. Provide an overview of the development of the food insecurity measure.
2. Discuss how the food security measure is currently constructed.
3. Describe the following food insecurity concepts: food security, food insecurity, low food security.
4. Describe the extent of food insecurity in the United States.
5. Understand how the food insecurity rate, food insecurity gap, and squared food insecurity gaps are constructed.

Key Terms

Core Food Security Module (CFSM): A measure of household food insecurity in the United States.

food insecurity: Occurs when some household members have limited or uncertain access to enough food because they lack resources for food.

food security: Occurs when all household members have access at all times to enough food for an active, healthy life.

very low food security: Occurs when one or more household members are hungry because they cannot afford enough food.

Introduction

Food insecurity in the United States has become a well-publicized issue of concern to policy makers and program administrators. More broadly, the extent of food insecurity is followed closely via media reports. The broad coverage of food insecurity is evidenced by, for example, a mention of the extent of food insecurity in an article in *Sports Illustrated* (Reilly, 2006). In 2005, 11.0% of the US population reported that they suffered from food insecurity at some time during the previous year (Nord, Andrews, & Carlson, 2006). For about 3.9% of the population, the degree of food insecurity was severe enough to be recorded as very low food security (formerly known as "food insecurity with hunger"). For households with children, the reported levels were higher: 15.6% and 4.1%, respectively.

In this chapter our first section consists of background about the food insecurity measure. This background consists of an overview of the development of the measure, followed by a description of how the food security measure is currently constructed. The second section contains descriptions of the extent of food insecurity in the United States. The third and final section reviews a new method of measuring food insecurity, which allows one to measure both the depth and severity of food insecurity.

Background

This section begins with a discussion of the history of the measurement of food insecurity. Following this is a comprehensive explanation of how food insecurity is measured.

History of the Measurement of Food Insecurity

Efforts leading to the current Core Food Security Module (CFSM) began in the early 1980s when President Reagan established the Task Force on Food Assistance to examine the food assistance programs and the claims of resurgence of hunger. After much investigative work, the task force made a distinction between two different working definitions of "hunger":

1. A scientific, clinical definition of hunger means "the actual physiological effects of extended nutritional deprivations."

2. A definition of hunger as commonly defined means "the inability, even occasionally, to obtain adequate food and nourishment" (US President, Task Force on Food Assistance, p. 34). The task force articulated the need for measuring hunger because there was no commonly accepted definition of hunger, much less its documentation at that time (National Research Council, 2006).

After the 1984 task force report, researchers in the private sector and government agencies increased their efforts to develop survey measures of the severity and extent of hunger in the United States. At this time, the main survey tool used to measure hunger was a single survey question on hunger. This question was the so-called food insufficiency question where respondents were asked the following question: *Which of these statements best describe the food eaten in your household in the last month?* Respondents have four choices: *enough of the kinds of food we want to eat, enough but not always the kinds of food we want to eat, sometimes not enough to eat,* or *often not enough to eat.* Going beyond this single question, the Food Research and Action Center (FRAC) sponsored a major series of surveys to study hunger among children (Radimer, Olson, & Campbell, 1990). A central component of these surveys was the development of food insecurity measures. This led, in 1990, to a report by the Life Sciences Research Office (LSRO) of the Federation of American Societies for Experimental Biology (FASEB). This report contains what have become the consensus conceptual definitions for the terms "food security," "food insecurity," and "hunger," as relevant to the United States, and notes the relationship of food insecurity to hunger and malnutrition (Anderson, 1990). The panel decided that redefining the hunger problem in terms of food security could overcome some of the earlier problems, including the seeming lack of a more objective measure (Anderson, 1990, p. 1575).

Using these LSRO conceptual definitions, the US Department of Agriculture (USDA) and the US Department of Health and Human Services (DHHS) began to develop operational definitions of food insecurity and hunger that are appropriate for use in large national population surveys. This move toward such measures was in response to Congress's enactment of the National Nutrition Monitoring and Related Research Act (NNMRR) (Public Law 101-445). In particular, Section 103 of the act required the preparation and implementation of a 10-year comprehensive plan to assess the dietary and nutritional status of the US population. Task V-C-2.4 in the plan specified (*Federal Register*, 1993, 58:32 752–806):

In 1992, USDA and HHS formed the Federal Food Security Measurement Project. This project brought together representatives from several federal agencies, academia, and private organizations. This interagency group developed the food security instrument, and the rules used to characterize the food security status of each household surveyed. This was followed, in 1994, with the USDA- and HHS-sponsored First National Conference on Food Security Measurement and Research. Numerous technical issues surfaced during this conference. In response, the USDA also commissioned additional analytical work based on two independent data sets on hunger and food insecurity: one developed at Cornell and the other by the Community Childhood Hunger Identification Project (CCHIP). We now turn to a discussion of the resulting food insecurity measure.

The Measurement of Food Insecurity

To calculate the official rates of food insecurity and food insecurity with hunger in the United States, a food security scale is constructed using a set of 18 questions for households with children and 10 questions for households without children. (The 10 questions are a subset of the 18.) Some of the conditions people are asked about include: "I worried whether our food would run out before we got money to buy more" (the least severe item), "Did you or the other adults in your household ever cut the size of your meals or skip meals because there wasn't enough money for food?" "Were you ever hungry but did not eat because you couldn't afford enough food?" and "Did a child in the household ever not eat for a full day because you couldn't afford enough food?" (the most severe item for households with children). (A complete list of questions is provided in Table 6.1.) Each of these questions is qualified by the proviso that the conditions are due to financial constraints. As a consequence, persons who have reduced food intakes due to, say, fasting for religious reasons or dieting, would not respond affirmatively to these questions. (The discussion in this section borrows heavily from Section 2.2 of Gundersen, 2008.)

These 18 questions are taken from a larger set of questions that were asked on the first CFSM in 1995. To narrow the set, questions

Table 6.1   Food Insecurity Questions in the Core Food Security Module

Food Insecurity Question	Households with Children		Households without Children	
	Number of affirmative responses	Rasch score	Number of affirmative responses	Rasch score
1. "We worried whether our food would run out before we got money to buy more." Was that **often**, **sometimes**, or never true for you in the last 12 months?	1	1.30	1	1.72
2. "The food that we bought just didn't last and we didn't have money to get more." Was that **often**, **sometimes**, or never true for you in the last 12 months?	2	2.56	23.10	
3. "We couldn't afford to eat balanced meals." Was that **often**, **sometimes**, or never true for you in the last 12 months?	3	3.41	3	4.23
4. "We relied on only a few kinds of low-cost food to feed our children because we were running out of money to buy food." Was that **often**, **sometimes**, or never true for you in the last 12 months?	4	4.14		
5. In the last 12 months, did you or other adults in the household ever cut the size of your meals or skip meals because there wasn't enough money for food? (**Yes**/No)	5	4.81	4	5.24

(continues)

Table 6.1   Food Insecurity Questions in the Core Food Security Module *(continued)*

Food Insecurity Question	Households with Children		Households without Children	
	Number of affirmative responses	Rasch score	Number of affirmative responses	Rasch score
6. "We couldn't feed our children a balanced meal, because we couldn't afford that." Was that **often**, **sometimes**, or never true for you in the last 12 months?	6	5.43		
7. In the last 12 months, did you ever eat less than you felt you should because there wasn't enough money for food? (**Yes**/No)	7	6.02	5	6.16
8. (If yes to Question 5) How often did this happen— **almost every month**, **some months but not every month**, or in only 1 or 2 months?	8	6.61	6	7.07
9. "The children were not eating enough because we just couldn't afford enough food." Was that **often**, **sometimes**, or never true for you in the last 12 months?	9	7.18		
10. In the last 12 months, were you ever hungry, but didn't eat, because you couldn't afford enough food? (**Yes**/No)	10	7.74	7	8.00

Food Insecurity Question	Households with Children		Households without Children	
	Number of affirmative responses	Rasch score	Number of affirmative responses	Rasch score
11. In the last 12 months, did you lose weight because you didn't have enough money for food? (**Yes**/No)	11	8.28	8	8.98
12. In the last 12 months, did you ever cut the size of any of the children's meals because there wasn't enough money for food? (**Yes**/No)	12	8.79		
13. In the last 12 months did you or other adults in your household ever not eat for a whole day because there wasn't enough money for food? (**Yes**/No)	13	9.31	9	10.15
14. In the last 12 months, were the children ever hungry but you just couldn't afford more food? (**Yes**/No)	14	9.84		
15. (If yes to Question 13) How often did this happen—**almost every month, some months but not every month**, or in only 1 or 2 months?	15	10.42	10	11.05
16. In the last 12 months, did any of the children ever skip a meal because there wasn't enough money for food? (**Yes**/No)	16	11.13		

(continues)

Table 6.1   Food Insecurity Questions in the Core Food Security Module *(continued)*

Food Insecurity Question	Households with Children		Households without Children	
	Number of affirmative responses	Rasch score	Number of affirmative responses	Rasch score
17. (If yes to Question 16) How often did this happen—**almost every month, some months but not every month,** or in only 1 or 2 months?	17	12.16		
18. In the last 12 months did any of the children ever not eat for a whole day because there wasn't enough money for food? (**Yes**/No)	18	13.03		

Notes: Responses in bold indicate an "affirmative" response. This is a modified version of a table taken from Gundersen, 2008.

that were deemed to be a poor fit with other questions were dropped from the scale. Conversely, questions that were deemed to be redundant with other questions were dropped from the scale. Along with being a good fit with the other questions and not being redundant, the 18 questions are considered to be a unidimensional representation of food insecurity. (For more on how the 18 questions were ultimately chosen and the justifications for these choices see Hamilton et al., 1997, especially Chapter 2.)

Learning Point: A household's food security status is defined by its answers to the questions on the Core Food Security Module.

Using the full set of 18 questions, the USDA delineates households into food insecurity categories subsequently described. The idea underlying the use of multiple questions is that no single question can accurately portray the concept of food insecurity. (An analogy can be drawn with the educational testing literature where the Rasch model is often used. In that case, it would be presumed that no one question can reflect a student's knowledge of, say, a particular subject, but rather a series of questions are needed to accurately portray his or her knowledge.) To map the 18 questions into food insecurity categories, the USDA first employs the Rasch model, a model that emerged out of the broader class of Item Response Theory models. (For more on Rasch scoring methods see, e.g., Andrich, 1988.)

> **Learning Point:** A Rasch model is used to map responses from a household's responses to the Core Food Security Module into its food insecurity status.

The results from estimating the Rasch model yield a value for each number of affirmative responses. These values can be seen as a reflection of the underlying severity of food insecurity that faces a household responding affirmatively to a particular number of questions.

The results of this Rasch score modeling for the official USDA measures can be seen in columns (2) and (4) in Table 6.1. These values range from 0 to 13.03 for households with children and from 0 to 11.05 for households without children. As can be seen, more affirmative responses to these questions are associated with higher Rasch scores and, thus, higher levels of food insecurity. To draw a parallel with income measures of well-being, more affirmative responses are equivalent to lower levels of income. In interpreting the values, one should note that the values are unique up to a linear transformation. Thus, the relative differences between the values matter, not the absolute differences. As an example, for households with children, responding affirmatively to 10 rather than nine questions raises the Rasch score by 0.56 while responding affirmatively to three rather than two questions raises it by 0.85. This would then imply that the severity of food insecurity increases more as one moves from two to three responses than from nine to 10 responses.

These Rasch scores are then used to establish the thresholds for:

(a) food security (i.e., cases where all household members had access at all times to enough food for an active, healthy life)
(b) low food security (i.e., cases where at least some household members were uncertain of having, or unable to acquire,

enough food because they had insufficient money and other resources for food)

(c) very low food security (i.e., cases where one or more household members were hungry, at least sometime during the year, because they couldn't afford enough food)

Categories (b) and (c) are often combined into the category of "food insecure." Households responding affirmatively to two or fewer questions are food secure; those responding to three to seven questions are defined as food insecure without hunger (three to five questions for households without children); and those responding to eight or more questions are defined as very low food secure (six or more for households without children). Consistent with the language employed in the literature, a household responding affirmatively to three or more questions is identified as food insecure. One should note that all households defined as very low food secure are also food insecure, but the converse is not true.

There are two other sets of food security categories used by researchers. The first is the so-called "marginal food insecurity" category. Under this definition, all households that respond affirmatively to one or more questions are defined as marginally food insecure. This is in contrast to the usual definition of food security previously described whereby households that respond affirmatively to one or two questions are defined as food secure. Note that all households in the food insecurity category are marginally food insecure, but the converse is not true. (For a use of this category see, e.g., Laraia, Siega-Riz, Gundersen, & Dole, 2006.)

The second set of food insecurity questions is defined with respect to children in a household. As a consequence, only the eight child-specific questions (i.e., those of the set of 18 questions that refer to the children in the household) are used. Under this measure, a household is said to be "child food insecure" if two or more questions are answered affirmatively and "very low child food secure" if five or more questions are answered affirmatively. (For uses of this measure see, e.g., Nord, 2003; Nord & Hopwood, 2007; Nord

> **Learning Point:** Researchers also use a further measure of food insecurity, the marginal food insecurity measure, and define food insecurity with respect to only the responses for the children in the household.

& Bickel, 2002; Connell, Lofton, Yadrick, & Rehner, 2005; Connell, Nord, Lofton, & Yadrick, 2004.)

Food Insecurity in the United States

In this section the extent of food insecurity is described for the United States from 2001 to 2005. Along with providing descriptions for (a) the full population, this is broken down into (b) households with children and (c) households without children. Because food insecurity is rare among households above 200% of the poverty line (Nord, et al., 2006), results along the lines of (a) through (c) are also displayed for households with incomes below this threshold. All of these are displayed in Figures 6.1 through 6.6.

These figures are calculated based on data from the Current Population Survey (CPS). More specifically, they are from the 2001 through 2005 December supplements from the CPS, a monthly survey of approximately 50,000 households. Along with being the official data source for official poverty and unemployment rates, in this supplement the CPS has the CFSM. The CFSM has been in at least 1 month in the CPS in every year since 1995. To avoid issues of seasonality and changes in various other things (e.g., the screening questions), only the five most recently available December supplements are used in these figures.

In every year from 2001 to 2005 about one in five Americans lived in households that experienced at least marginal food insecurity. For the more severe levels of food insecurity (food insecurity and very low food security), the figures are about 10% to 12% and 3% to 4%. The figures remain relatively constant across all 5 years for each of the categories.

When one looks at households with children, the picture is worse. As seen in Figure 6.2, from 2001 to 2005, about one in four households with children experienced at least marginal food insecurity. The more severe levels of food insecurity were also higher among households with children—over 15% of households with children were food insecure and almost 5% were very low food secure. For households without children, the food insecurity numbers are better than for the population as a whole. This can be seen in Figure 6.3.

In Figures 6.4 through 6.6, we restrict our attention to households with incomes below 200% of the poverty line. Because households with

FIGURE 6.1   Food Insecurity Rates, 2001 to 2005

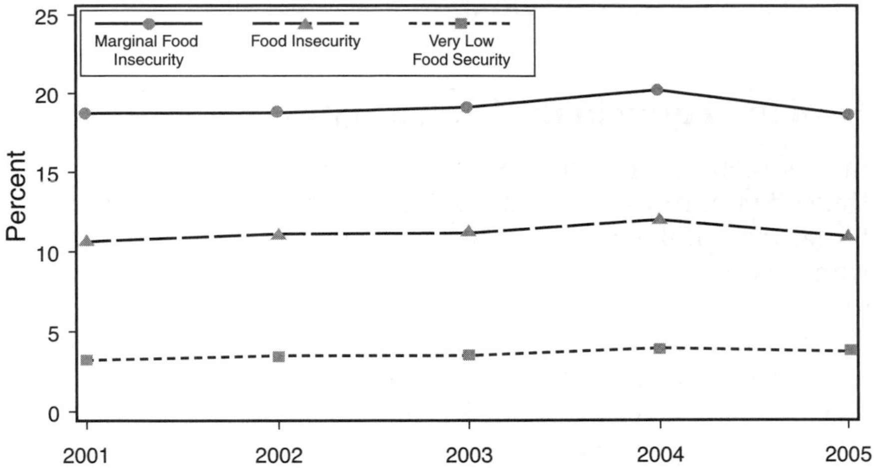

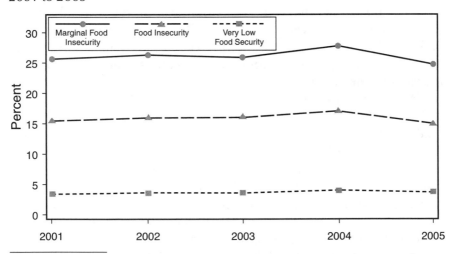

Source: Calculations by Gundersen based on data from the 2001 to 2005 Current Population
Survey.

lower incomes are more prone to being food insecure, as expected,
the proportion of households that suffer from food insecurity is
higher than the corresponding results in Figures 6.1 through 6.3. For

FIGURE 6.2   Food Insecurity Rates, Households with Children,
2001 to 2005

Source: Calculations by Gundersen based on data from the 2001 to 2005 Current Population
Survey.

FIGURE 6.3   Food Insecurity Rates, Households without Children, 2001 to 2005

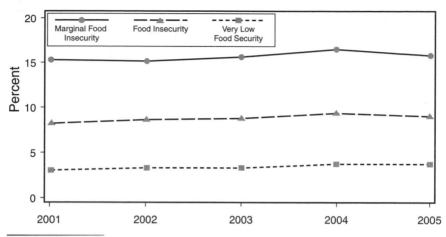

Source: Calculations by Gundersen based on data from the 2001 to 2005 Current Population Survey.

the US population whose incomes were less than 200% of the poverty line, on average, more than 42% reported experiencing some level of food insecurity during the previous year (Figure 6.4). The

FIGURE 6.4   Food Insecurity Rates, Incomes <200% of the Poverty Line, 2001 to 2005

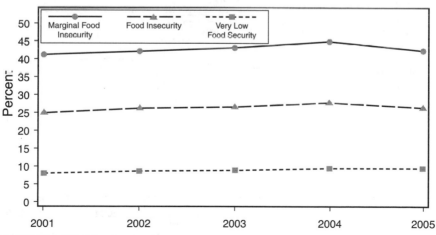

Source: Calculations by Gundersen based on data from the 2001 to 2005 Current Population Survey.

FIGURE 6.5   Food Insecurity Rates, Incomes <200% of the Poverty Line, Households with Children, 2001 to 2005

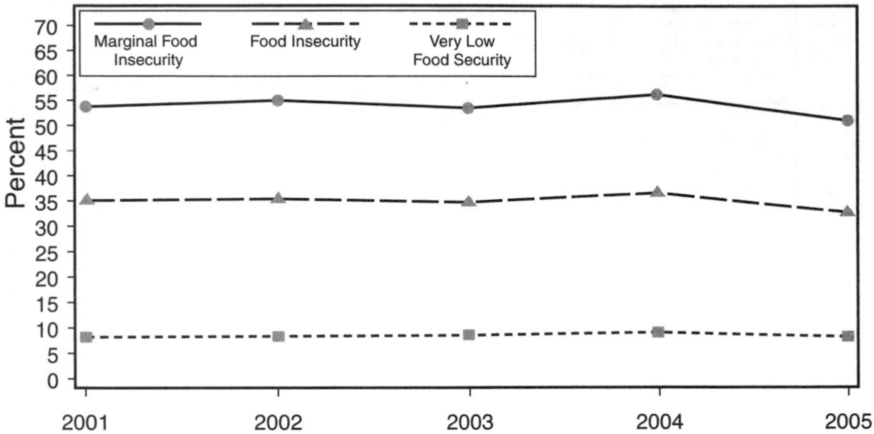

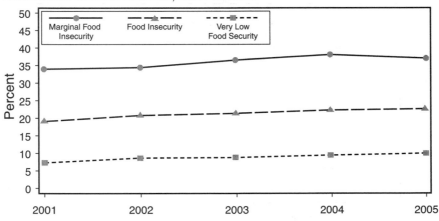

Source: Calculations by Gundersen based on data from the 2001 to 2005 Current Population Survey.

average percentages for households both with and without children were also higher: 54% and 34%, respectively (Figures 6.5 and 6.6). Food insecurity levels were, on average, 26% for the full population

FIGURE 6.6   Food Insecurity Rates, Incomes <200% of the Poverty Line, Households without Children, 2001 to 2005

Source: Calculations by Gundersen based on data from the 2001 to 2005 Current Population Survey.

of households with incomes below 200% of the poverty line, 34% for households with children with incomes below 200% of the poverty line, and 22% for households without children with incomes below 200% of the poverty line.

Measuring the Extent, Depth, and Severity of Food Insecurity in the United States

The methods used to describe food insecurity in the United States described in the previous sections are clear and straightforward. However, when these binary comparisons are used (e.g., food insecure versus not food insecure), a great deal of information is being suppressed. In particular, information is not being utilized when broad categories are created from the 18 questions on the CFSM. As an example, consider two households, one responding affirmatively to eight questions and one responding affirmatively to 18 questions. Both are treated as very low food secure yet, arguably, the latter household has a higher level of food insecurity. This section describes a set of measures that portray the extent, depth, and severity of food insecurity. Along with utilizing more of the information contained in the CFSM, this series of measures allow one to ascertain the robustness of comparisons of food insecurity between groups. (These measures were first established for food insecurity in Dutta & Gundersen, 2007.)

> **Learning Point:** The methods used to describe food insecurity in the United States seem to be clear and straightforward. However, when these binary comparisons are used (e.g., food insecure versus not food insecure), a great deal of information is being suppressed.

The three measures are described as follows:

$$d^0 = \frac{q}{n} \qquad \text{food insecurity rate}$$

$$d^1 = \frac{\sum_{i=1}^{q} d_i}{n} \qquad \text{food insecurity gap}$$

$$d^2 = \frac{\sum_{i=1}^{q} d_i}{n} \qquad \text{squared food insecurity gap}$$

where q is the number of food insecure households, n is the total number of households, and d_i is the level of food insecurity for a household i.

An application of this broader set of measures to the food insecurity status of American Indians and non-American Indians can be found in Tables 6.2 (all households) and 6.3 (households with incomes below 185% of the poverty line). Akin to the information in Figures 6.1 through 6.6, these tables are derived from data in the CPS from the years 2001 to 2004. (These tables are modified versions of those found in Gundersen, 2008.)

Table 6.2   Food Insecurity for American Indians and Non-American Indians

Food insecurity measure	American Indians	Non-American Indians	Ratio of columns (1) and (2)
Households with children			
Food insecurity rate ($\alpha = 0$)	0.280**	0.157	1.783
	(0.020)	(0.002)	
Food insecurity gap ($\alpha = 1$)	0.077**	0.041	1.878
	(0.007)	(0.001)	
Squared food insecurity gap ($\alpha = 2$)	0.030**	0.015	2.000
	(0.004)	(0.0004)	
Households without children			
Food insecurity rate ($\alpha = 0$)	0.163**	0.078	2.090
	(0.013)	(0.001)	
Food insecurity gap ($\alpha = 1$)	0.081**	0.031	2.613
	(0.008)	(0.001)	
Squared food insecurity gap ($\alpha = 2$)	0.053**	0.018	2.944
	(0.006)	(0.0003)	

Data are from the 2001 to 2004 Current Population Survey. Standard errors are in parentheses. Superscripts of ** are used in column (1) if the p-value of the difference between columns (1) and (2) is less than 0.05 or 0.01, respectively.

Source: Gundersen, 2008.

Table 6.3 Food Insecurity for American Indians and Non-American Indians, Households with Incomes Below 185% of the Poverty Line

Food insecurity measure	American Indians	Non-American Indians	Ratio of columns (1) and (2)
Households with children			
Food insecurity rate ($\alpha = 0$)	0.417*	0.348	1.198
	(0.030)	(0.005)	
Food insecurity gap ($\alpha = 1$)	0.120*	0.093	1.290
	(0.011)	(0.002)	
Squared food insecurity gap ($\alpha = 2$)	0.047*	0.035	1.343
	(0.006)	(0.001)	
Households without children			
Food insecurity rate ($\alpha = 0$)	0.305**	0.191	1.597
	(0.026)	(0.003)	
Food insecurity gap ($\alpha = 1$)	0.158**	0.080	1.975
	(0.017)	(0.002)	
Squared food insecurity gap ($\alpha = 2$)	0.105**	0.047	2.234
	(0.013)	(0.001)	

Data are from the 2001 to 2004 Current Population Survey. Standard errors are in parentheses. Superscripts of * or ** are used in column (1) if the p-value of the difference between columns (1) and (2) is less than 0.05 or 0.01, respectively.

Source: Gundersen, 2008.

Across all three measures (food insecurity rate, food insecurity gap, squared food insecurity gap), food insecurity is higher among American Indians than among non-American Indians, and these differences are statistically significant. This is true for both households with and without children. These differences are not all that surprising. American Indians have per capita incomes that are 40% less than the entire population (Leichenko, 2003); large numbers of American Indians have earnings in the lower end of the income distribution (Gregory, Abello, & Johnson, 1997); and counties with a high proportion of American Indians have lower incomes than counties with low proportions of American Indians (Leichenko, 2003, Table 6.2). Thus, the orderings (i.e., whether American Indians or non-American Indians have higher levels of food insecurity) are robust to at least these three food insecurity measures. Similar results hold for the low-income sample of Table 6.3.

Along with considering whether American Indians have higher food insecurity than non-American Indians across the three measures, one might also wonder whether the magnitude of the differences is similar across the measures. One way to consider this is by taking the ratio of the food insecurity measures for American Indians to non-American Indians. These results are in column (3) of Tables 6.2 and 6.3.

For the sample of households with children, the ratios are quite similar across all three measures for both all households and for the low-income sample. For the sample of households without children, however, the ratios differ markedly as more weight is placed on the food insecurity of those with higher food insecurity levels (i.e., as the value of α increases). For the all-income sample of households without children, the ratio is 2.09 when $\alpha = 0$, and it is 2.94 when $\alpha = 2$. For the low-income sample, the figures are 1.60 and 2.23. So, in households with children, the conclusions one draws regarding differences between American Indians and non-American Indians depend on the choice of food security measure.

Chapter Summary

In response to concerns about hunger in the United States, a series of studies were undertaken to measure hunger in the United States and ascertain its extent. This led to the development of the Core Food Security Module (CFSM). With the CFSM, the extent of hunger in the United States has been established and is presented in a closely followed series of annual reports. Approximately one in five Americans experiences some degree of food insecurity with substantially higher rates for households with children and for households with low incomes. Recent work has used the CFSM to establish a wider array of food insecurity measures.

Issues to Debate

1. Discuss why we should (or should not) be concerned about food insecurity in the United States.

2. Discuss what sorts of policies the United States might wish to pursue to help alleviate food insecurity.
3. Discuss possible reasons for why households with children have higher rates of food insecurity than those without children.

References

Anderson, S. (1990). Core indicators of nutritional state for difficult-to-sample populations. *Journal of Nutrition, 120*, 1559S–1600S.

Andrich, D. (1988). *Rasch models for measurement*. Newbury Park, CA: Sage Publications.

Connell, C., Lofton, K., Yadrick, K., & Rehner, T. (2005). Children's experiences of food insecurity can assist in understanding its effect on their well-being. *Journal of Nutrition, 135*, 1683–1690.

Connell, C., Nord, M., Lofton, K., & Yadrick, K. (2004). Food security of older children can be assessed using a standardized survey instrument. *Journal of Nutrition, 134*, 2566–2572.

Dutta, I., & Gundersen, C. (2007). Measures of food insecurity at the household level. In B. Guha-Khasnobis, B. Acharya, & B. Davis (Eds.), *Food security indicators, measurement, and the impact of trade openness: Series: WIDER studies in development economics*. Oxford, England: Oxford University Press.

Gregory, R., Abello, A., & Johnson, J. (1997). The individual economic well-being of Native American men and women during the 1980s: A decade of moving backwards. *Population Research and Policy Review, 16*, 115–145.

Gundersen, C. (2008). Measuring the extent, depth, and severity of food insecurity: An application to American Indians in the United States. *Journal of Population Economics, 21*(1), 191–215.

Hamilton, W., Cook, J., Thompson, W., Burn, L., Frongillo, E., Olson, C., et al. (1997). *Household food security in the United States in 1995: Technical report of the food security measurement project*. Alexandria, VA: US Department of Agriculture, Food and Consumer Service, Office of Analysis and Evaluation.

Laraia, B., Siega-Riz, A., Gundersen, C., & Dole, N. (2006). Psychosocial factors and socioeconomic indicators are associated with household food insecurity among pregnant women. *Journal of Nutrition, 136*, 177–182.

Leichenko, R. (2003). Does place still matter? Accounting for income variation across American Indian tribal areas. *Economic Geography, 79*, 365–386.

National Research Council. (2006). *Food insecurity and hunger in the United States: An assessment of the measure*. Washington, DC: National Academies Press.

Nord, M. (2003). *Food insecurity in households with children* (Food Assistance and Nutrition Research Report No. 34-13). Washington, DC: US Department of Agriculture, Economic Research Service.

Nord, M., Andrews, M., & Carlson, S. (2006). *Household food security in the United States, 2005* (Economic Research Report No. 29). Washington, DC: US Department of Agriculture, Economic Research Service.

Nord, M., & Bickel, G. (2002). *Measuring children's food security in US households, 1995-1999* (Food Assistance and Nutrition Research Report No. 25). Washington, DC: US Department of Agriculture, Economic Research Service.

Nord, M., & Hopwood, H. (2007). Recent advances provide improved tools for measuring children's food security. *Journal of Nutrition, 137,* 533-536.

Radimer, K., Olson, C., & Campbell, C. (1990). Development of indicators to assess hunger. *Journal of Nutrition, 120,* 1544-1548.

Reilly, R. (2006). A bone to pick with Boone. *Sports Illustrated, 114.*

US President, Task Force on Food Assistance. (1984). *Report of the President's Task Force on Food Assistance.* Washington, DC: US Government Printing Office.

CHAPTER 7

THE DETERMINANTS OF FOOD INSECURITY IN THE UNITED STATES

Craig Gundersen, PhD

Chapter Objectives

After reading the chapter and reflecting on the contents, you should be able to:

1. Provide an overview of factors that might contribute to whether a household is food insecure.
2. Explain what types of households are most likely to be at risk for food insecurity.
3. Discuss the major characteristics of food insecure households.
4. Understand how the life cycle model helps to explain food insecurity.
5. Understand the dynamic nature of determinants of food insecurity.

Key Terms

determinant: A variable that can be used to predict or explain another variable.
food security mobility: The ability of households and/or individuals to move from one food security level to another.
life cycle model: Shows how different stages in an individual's life are related to his or her level of food security.
multivariate analysis: Allows a researcher to examine the relationship between two variables while controlling the effects of other variables.
panel survey: A study of the same group of people over time.

state food security infrastructure: Several types of characteristics that have been shown to be related to household food security that varies by state.

Introduction

The previous chapter demonstrated why food insecurity is of concern to policy makers and program administrators. While about one in 10 Americans are food insecure, the proportion increases when one examines households with incomes below 200% of the poverty line. Along with low income, there are numerous other factors that help to determine whether a household is food insecure. In this chapter we portray these other factors.

The first section of this chapter presents summary statistics, in a series of bar graphs, about the prevalence of food insecurity among various categories. This will give the reader some sense as to what types of households are most likely to be at risk of food insecurity. The second section reviews the evidence regarding the major determinants of food insecurity, controlling for other factors.

Characteristics of the Food Insecure in the United States

In this section the characteristics of the food insecure population are described for the United States. We do so in Figures 7.1–7.11 where we display the proportion within any category (e.g., homeowners) that is (1) marginally food secure, (2) food insecure, or (3) low food secure. For data, we use information from the 2001 to 2005 Current Population Survey, the same data used in Chapter 6. We combine all 5 years for the analyses to ensure large enough sample sizes.

As seen in Figure 7.1, when one looks at households by income categories, the level of food insecurity occurs in 39% of families with incomes at or below the poverty line. For families whose income falls between 100% and 200% of the poverty line, this figure drops to 20%.

The second category used to describe the food insecure population is race/ethnicity. Figures 7.2 and 7.3 distinguish the household food insecurity rates by racial categories. The level of food insecurity markedly differed in its occurrence in households headed by either an

FIGURE 7.1   Food Insecurity Rates by Income Categories

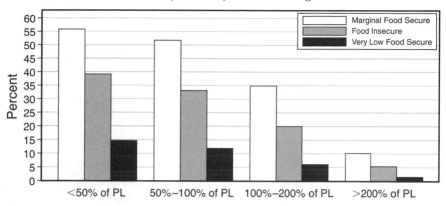

Source: Calculations by Gundersen based on data from the 2001 to 2005 Current Population Survey.

African American or Hispanic American person as compared to households headed by a white person—23%, 21%, and 9%, respectively.

Other categories used to describe food insecurity rates are marital status, home ownership, and metropolitan status. Figure 7.4 shows that over one in four never married households have experienced food insecurity, while less than one in seven divorced or separated households have experienced food insecurity. There is a

FIGURE 7.2   Food Insecurity Rates by Racial Categories

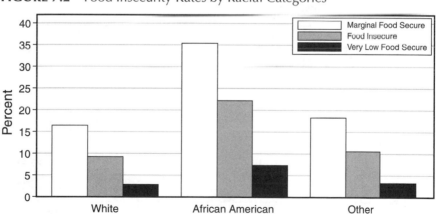

Source: Calculations by Gundersen based on data from the 2001 to 2005 Current Population Survey.

FIGURE 7.3   Food Insecurity Rates by Hispanic Categories

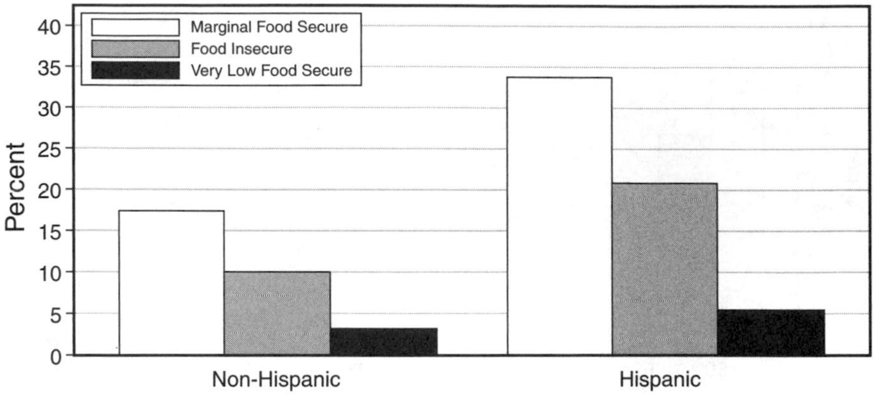

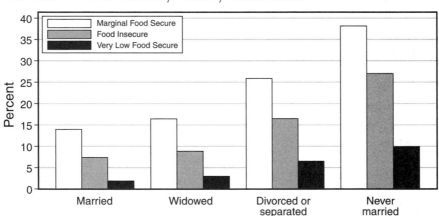

Source: Calculations by Gundersen based on data from the 2001 to 2005 Current Population Survey.

dramatic drop in food insecurity levels among married and widowed households—7% and 9%, respectively. Similar differences are also seen between the homeowner and non-homeowner status groups in Figure 7.5. While 20% of non-homeowner households had experienced food insecurity, only 6% of homeowner households had experienced food insecurity. As shown in Figure 7.6, food insecurity rates were more similar when viewed by metropolitan status—metropolitan households, 11%; nonmetropolitan households, 12%.

FIGURE 7.4   Food Insecurity Rates by Marital Status

Source: Calculations by Gundersen based on data from the 2001 to 2005 Current Population Survey.

FIGURE 7.5 Food Insecurity Rates by Home Ownership Status

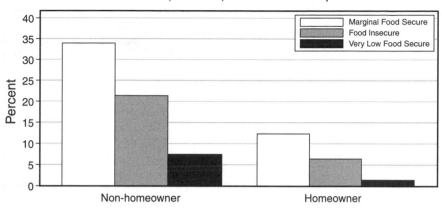

Source: Calculations by Gundersen based on data from the 2001 to 2005 Current Population Survey.

More characteristics by which food insecurity rates are examined include age of household head, employment of household head, and region of country. As seen in Figure 7.7, as the age of the household head increases from less than 30 years to 30–50 years, to 50–70 years, and to more than 70 years, the levels of food insecurity drop from 17%, 13%, 8%, and 5%, respectively. Figure 7.8 shows the influence of employment status of household head on food insecurity. While 30% of unemployed status households are food insecure, less than

FIGURE 7.6 Food Insecurity Rates by Metropolitan Status

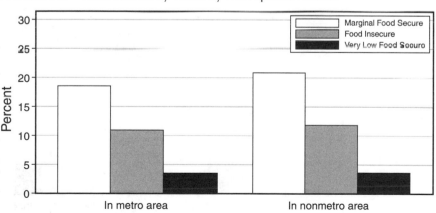

Source: Calculations by Gundersen based on data from the 2001 to 2005 Current Population Survey.

FIGURE 7.7   Food Insecurity Rates by Age of Household Head

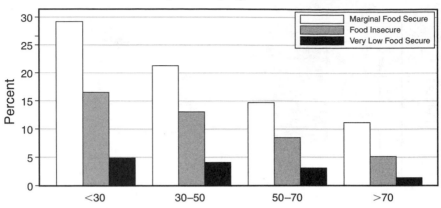

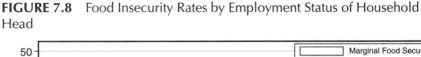

Source: Calculations by Gundersen based on data from the 2001 to 2005 Current Population Survey.

10% of employed households are food insecure. Nearly 25% of disabled status households are food insecure. However, only 5% of retired status households are categorized as food insecure. Figure 7.9 shows the differences in food insecurity rates by region (Northeast, Midwest, South, West). As seen, the rates are similar in the Northeast and Midwest but are higher in the South and West. These comparisons hold across all three measures.

FIGURE 7.8   Food Insecurity Rates by Employment Status of Household Head

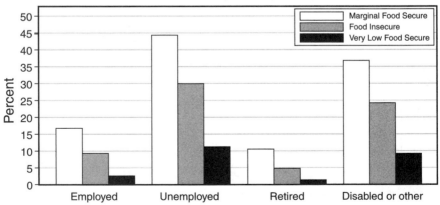

Source: Calculations by Gundersen based on data from the 2001 to 2005 Current Population Survey.

FIGURE 7.9   Food Insecurity Rates by Region of Country

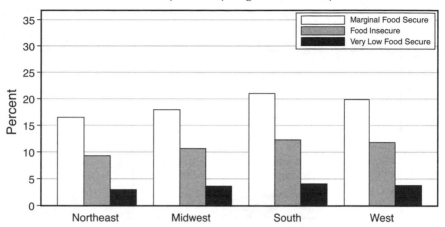

Source: Calculations by Gundersen based on data from the 2001 to 2005 Current Population Survey.

Finally, food insecurity has been linked to the education level of the household head and the presence of children in the household, as shown in Figures 7.10 and 7.11, respectively. As the education

FIGURE 7.10   Food Insecurity Rates by Education Level of Household Head

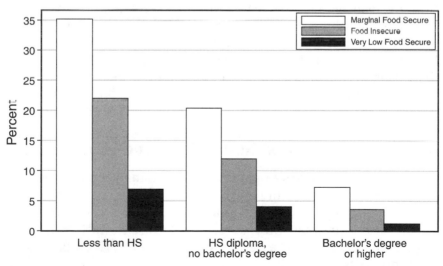

Source: Calculations by Gundersen based on data from the 2001 to 2005 Current Population Survey.

FIGURE 7.11   Food Insecurity Rates by Presence of Children

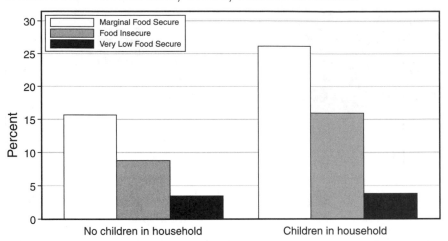

Source: Calculations by Gundersen based on data from the 2001 to 2005 Current Population Survey.

Learning Point: Food insecurity is linked to a variety of factors.

---

level of the household head increases, the percentage of households that are food insecure decreases, from 23% for households whose head has less than a high school degree to 4% for households whose head has at least a bachelor's degree. Similarly, the percentage of households with food insecurity changes with the presence of children, from 9% to households without children to 16% for households with children.

Determinants of Food Insecurity in the United States

We now turn to a series of papers that have analyzed the determinants of food insecurity in the United States. These papers have appeared in a wide variety of journals across a wide variety of disciplines. Moreover, they use many different statistical techniques and data sets to ascertain the effect of various factors on food insecurity.

Dynamic Determinants of Food Insecurity

Policy makers and social scientists are interested in understanding the processes that generate economic hardship in US households. Studies have found that poverty can be persistent, with poor families being more likely than non-poor families to be poor in the future. Although researchers have investigated poverty, relatively less research has been conducted on consumption-based hardships such as food insecurity. (An exception is Gundersen & Gruber, 2001.)

Ribar and Hamrick (2003) compared the dynamics of poverty and food insecurity using longitudinal data from the 1993 panel of the Survey of Income and Program Participation (SIPP) and the Survey of Program Dynamics (SPD) in the context of a life cycle model of income and food consumption. This study is unique in two ways. First, it analyzes whether food problems are relatively short or long lasting by assessing whether people who experience them are more likely to experience food problems in the future and whether different groups of people have distinct patterns of food security mobility. Second, this study considers whether poverty and food insecurity are distinct manifestations of the same process.

With this longitudinal data set, the authors found new insights into the dynamics of food insecurity. Persistence in food insecurity was low, with 79% of the initial households with food problems at the start of the study having no problems 2 years later. While this holds for the full population, subsamples do differ. For example, multivariate analysis found that female-headed households are especially prone to being food insecure. Furthermore, low levels of income, which is an indicator of a household's ability to spread out consumption costs over time, are also associated with food problems.

> **Learning Point:** Longitudinal data give new insights into the dynamics of food insecurity.

State-Level Determinants of Food Insecurity

Extensive research has been conducted on the determinants of food insecurity using household-level data. (In addition to the papers discussed in this chapter, see, e.g., Dunifon & Kowaleski-Jones, 2003;

Bhattacharya, Currie, & Haider, 2004; Borjas, 2004; Furness, Simon, Wold, & Asarian-Anderson, 2004; Bitler, Gundersen, & Marquis, 2005; Van Hook & Balistreri, 2006; and Gundersen, 2008.) Much less research has been done using data aggregated to the state level.

An exception is Bartfeld and Dunifon (2006). To further the understanding of the relationships between specific state characteristics and food insecurity, Bartfeld and Dunifon examined interstate variation in household food security levels. While some of the predictors of food insecurity will be similar between states, each state with its accompanying "state food security infrastructure" will both directly influence and moderate the level of availability, accessibility, and affordability of household food-related needs.

Within these state food security infrastructures, there are three main reasons why predictors of food insecurity might be different between states. First, federal assistance programs, such as the Food Stamp Program and the National School Breakfast and Lunch Programs, have criteria that are similar across the country. However, states differ in other criteria, including vehicle restrictions, frequency of recertification, location of the application sites, and job search requirements. Second, tax policies that affect financial resources of low-income households are an important component of the state food security infrastructure. States differ on their dependence on income, property, and sales taxes, which, in turn, have repercussions for low-income households. Third, states with more favorable economic conditions, such as availability of quality jobs, cost of living, and social connections among community members, would be expected to have lower levels of food insecurity.

The authors used data from the 1998 through 2001 Core Food Security Module (CFSM) on the Current Population Survey (CPS). The data were supplemented with state-level data that described various facets of the food security infrastructure. With this data, the authors used hierarchical modeling in which both household-level and state-level characteristics are thought to affect food security outcomes. The following several state-level characteristics appeared to be linked with household food insecurity: the availability and accessibility of federal nutrition assistance programs, state-level tax policies, and states' economic and social characteristics. The authors found that a strong food security infrastructure is especially beneficial to families that are economically vulnerable even though they have incomes above the poverty line.

> **Learning Point:** Public policies can influence the extent of food insecurity within a state.

Effects of Income and Work Changes on Food Insecurity

Welfare recipients constitute a population that is often in danger of being food insecure, and these troubles often continue, even after leaving the welfare system. Despite the numerous studies of welfare recipients, little is known about what influences whether a current or past recipient of Temporary Assistance for Needy Families (TANF) experiences food insecurity. Along with the usual determinants of food insecurity, many TANF recipients' physical limitations and mental health problems are at a higher level than the general population.

In their study, Heflin, Corcoran, and Siefert (2007) examined the determinants of food insecurity. Along with looking at the usual determinants and physical and mental health limitations, they also used a panel survey such that they were able to control for unobserved heterogeneity. This study investigated determinants of changes in food insecurity status over time within a Michigan welfare sample using five waves of the Women's Employment Study (WES)—a panel survey that examined barriers to employment among mothers who were receiving cash assistance from TANF.

The authors found that hours worked, transportation expenses, and measures of coping ability are associated with food insecurity without controlling for unobservable differences. However, after using conditional fixed-effect logistic regression models, having at least one mental health problem and a low level of financial resources were the only determinants that remained associated with food insecurity.

Social Capital and Food Insecurity

Several studies have shown associations between social capital and positive individual and community outcomes. However, research on the effect of social capital on food insecurity is more limited. An exception is Martin, Rogers, Cook, and Joseph (2004, p. 2645), who examined the association between "social capital—a measure of trust, reciprocity, and social networks" and household food insecurity.

Using a cross-sectional design, door-to-door interviews were conducted with households that had incomes below 185% of the poverty line, targeting households at risk of food insecurity. Logistic regression models were used to determine if social capital at both the household and community levels significantly decreases the chances of being food insecure. Results showed that social capital at household and community levels is associated with decreased risk of food insecurity even after controlling for household income, education, and the employment status of adult members.

Food Insecurity among the Homeless

Along with food insecurity, another serious public health issue in the United States is homelessness. On any given day, at least 800,000 people in the United States might experience a period of homelessness and, at some point in the previous year, as many as 3.5 million people experience a period of homelessness (Burt & Aron, 2001). Homelessness is of particular concern for families with children. Over 1 million children are homeless in the course of a year (Burt & Aron, 2001).

Insofar as the determinants of homelessness and food insecurity are similar (e.g., low income, less education, single parenthood), one expects that families at higher risk of homelessness will also be food insecure. However, when we control for these observed characteristics, the relationship is not as transparent.

On the one hand, families who seek to maintain food security might be willing to accept a higher propensity to be homeless. For example, these families might forego payments of rent or mortgages to have enough food to eat (Kim, Ohls, & Cohen, 2001). By foregoing these payments, the likelihood of a possible eviction will increase. If this is the case, families with a higher propensity to homelessness, ceteris paribus, might have lower food insecurity levels. Similarly, a family with a strong taste for food consumption might endure homelessness rather than cutting back on food. On the other hand, a higher propensity to be homeless might be associated with higher levels of food insecurity. As an example, a family might accept a higher probability of homelessness to maintain consumption of other goods (e.g., medical care for a sick child). In the process of maintaining consumption of other goods, there might be a coincident decrease in food consumption. Or, because higher propensities to homelessness presumably also lead to greater stress levels, this might impair a mother's ability to successfully feed her family.

Gundersen, Weinreb, Wehler, and Hosmer (2003) analyze the relationship between the propensity toward homelessness and food insecurity using a sample of low-income housed and homeless women with children in Worcester, Massachusetts. This data set is unique in three ways. First, it has information on homeless families. This is the first time the determinants of food insecurity have been analyzed in a sample of homeless families, a group presumably at high risk of food insecurity. Second, the data set has information on housed low-income families as well. This gives us a comparison group to identify the effect of homelessness on food insecurity. Third, it has extensive information about the histories of the mothers, the mothers' and children's current medical conditions and their use of medical services, the social networks available to families, and the mothers' coping strategies. Previous work on samples restricted to low-income households has noted the lack of correlation of usual socioeconomic variables with food insecurity in multivariate models; with this data set we are able to consider a richer set of variables.

With this data set and an instrumental variables model, the authors find that families with mothers in better general health, families with infants, and families with mothers who have siblings who can provide monetary assistance are less likely to be food insecure. Conversely, mothers who were sexually abused as children are more likely to be food insecure. Within some of the models, homeless families are more likely to be food insecure, but in other models the effect is statistically insignificant.

Food Insecurity among Pregnant Women

One group of particular concern to policy makers are households with a pregnant woman. While some of the predictors of food insecurity will be similar with this group and other groups, there are three main reasons why predictors of food insecurity might be different for this population. First, the nutrient demands of pregnant women differ from that of non-pregnant women, with suggested increased intakes of most vitamins and minerals, and an additional 1.256 kj per day on average for a woman of normal weight (Institute of Medicine, 2002). To achieve optimal gestational weight gain, dietary requirements include nutrient-dense foods that are often more expensive (Drewnowski & Specter, 2004). At a minimum, purchasing food to increase a woman's daily caloric intake by 1.256 kj means the household faces more constraints in their food budget. To address these problems during pregnancy, federal food programs such as WIC might be available to low-income women; however, the Food Stamp Program (a program with far higher monthly monetary benefits in comparison to WIC) does not increase benefit levels until after a child is born. (See Chapter 9 for more information on WIC and the Food Stamp Program.)

Second, a pregnant woman might have more difficulty putting forth the effort to make nutritious food purchases. In response, someone other than the pregnant woman might make food purchases. If this person is less experienced in food shopping, this might lead to purchases that are less nutritious; if this person is also less experienced in food preparation, more expensive purchases (e.g., fast food) might be made. These two factors together can strain a household's food budget.

Third, a woman might exit the workforce during her pregnancy, decreasing the amount of money available for food. A sudden decrease can also present challenges to households that are not used to budgeting on a lower income (Gundersen & Gruber, 2001; Ribar & Hamrick, 2003). While food stamps can help a family's financial situation, applying for and receiving food stamps is not an instantaneous process.

To see how the determinants of food insecurity might differ for pregnant women, Laraia, Siega-Riz, Gundersen, and Dole (2006) examined data taken from the Pregnancy, Infection, and Nutrition (PIN) cohort, a prospective study that examines the influence of infection, physical activity, nutrition, food security, and stress on preterm birth. Between 2000 and 2004, 1510 women were recruited through the University of North Carolina Hospitals residents' and private physicians' obstetrics clinics before 20 weeks' gestation. With these data, the authors considered the effects of the standard set of factors (e.g., income, race/ethnicity) along with several psychosocial measures. These measures were as follows: Cohen's Perceived Stress Scale, Spielberger's Trait Anxiety Inventory, the Center for Epidemiologic Studies Depression (CES-D) Scale, Rosenberg's Self Esteem Scale, Pearlin's Mastery Scale, and Levenson's IPC Locus of Control with three subscales: the Internality Scale, the Powerful Others Scale, and the Chances Scale. (For more details about these measures see Laraia et al., 2006.)

After controlling for other factors, income, maternal age, and race were all predictors of household food insecurity. In addition, the psychosocial measures affected a household's probability of being food insecure. In particular, their measure of depressive symptoms was associated with household food insecurity.

> **Learning Point:** The reasons for food insecurity among pregnant women can differ slightly from other groups.

Determinants of Food Insecurity among the Elderly

Although many studies have examined food insecurity, understanding its nature and prevalence among the elderly is becoming increasingly important as this segment of the US population dramatically increases throughout the next decades. One gap in understanding the nature of food insecurity among the elderly is that the current concept of food insecurity has not taken into account the limited or uncertain food use among the elderly due to their functional impairments and health problems. According to Lee and Frongillo (2001, p. S94), food use "is the ability to prepare, gain access to, and eat food that is available in the household."

To see how the determinants of food insecurity among the elderly can differ, the authors examined data from the Third National Health and Nutrition Examination Survey (NHANES III) in New York state. Data were taken from 553 elderly persons having characteristics that reflect the US population. With these data, the authors considered the standard set of factors (e.g., income, race/ethnicity, educational level, age, and food assistance program participation) along with two categories of physical functioning activities. These categories were activities of daily living (ADL), such as dressing, eating, and getting in or out of a chair/bed, and instrumental activities of daily living (IADL), such as getting around by car, managing money, and taking medications. Low income, low education, minority status, food assistance program participation, and social isolation were all related to food insecurity. Even after controlling for other factors, functional impairments were related to food insecurity.

Chapter Summary

In response to concerns about food insecurity in the United States, several studies have been undertaken to determine the major factors that are associated with a household's food security level. In addition to low income levels, research has shown that several other characteristics are associated with higher levels of food insecurity. After controlling for other factors, major determinants of food insecurity have been found, which help to explain why food insecurity exists in the United States.

Issues to Debate

1. Discuss how the previously discussed determinants of food insecurity may or may not be interrelated and the possible reasons for the interrelatedness or lack of interrelatedness.
2. Discuss what sorts of policies the United States might wish to pursue to alleviate food insecurity based on the information learned thus far.
3. Discuss examples of cases where public policy might not be able to be changed to have any influence on food insecurity.

References

Bartfeld, J., & Dunifon, R. (2006). State-level predictor of food insecurity among households with children. *Journal of Policy Analysis and Management, 25,* 921–942.

Bhattacharya, J., Currie, J., & Haider, S. (2004). Poverty, food insecurity, and nutritional outcomes in children and adults. *Journal of Health Economics, 23*(4), 839–862.

Bitler, M., Gundersen, C., & Marquis, G. (2005). Are WIC non-recipients at less nutritional risk than recipients? An application of the food security measure. *Review of Agricultural Economics, 27*(3), 433–438.

Borjas, G. (2004). Food insecurity and public assistance. *Journal of Public Economics, 88*(7–8), 1421–1443.

Burt, M., & Aron, L. (2001). *Helping America's homeless.* Washington, DC: Urban Institute.

Drewnowski, A., & Specter, S. E. (2004). Poverty and obesity: The role of energy density and energy costs. *American Journal of Clinical Nutrition, 79,* 6–16.

Dunifon, R., & Kowaleski-Jones, L. (2003). The influences of participation in the National School Lunch Program and food insecurity on child well-being. *Social Service Review, 77*(1), 72–92.

Furness, B., Simon, P., Wold, C., & Asarian-Anderson, J. (2004). Prevalence and predictors of food insecurity among low-income households in Los Angeles County. *Public Health Nutrition, 7*(6), 791–794.

Gundersen, C. (2008). Measuring the extent, depth, and severity of food insecurity: An application to American Indians in the United States. *Journal of Population Economics, 21*(1), 191–215.

Gundersen, C., & Gruber, J. (2001). The dynamic predictors of food insufficiency. In M. Andrews & M. Prell (Eds.), *Second food security measurement and research conference, volume II: Papers* (pp. 92–110). US Department of Agriculture, Economic Research Service, Food Assistance and Nutrition Research Report 11-2.

Gundersen, C., Weinreb, L., Wehler, C., & Hosmer., D. (2003). Homelessness and food insecurity. *Journal of Housing Economics, 12*, 250–272.

Heflin, C., Corcoran, M., & Siefert, K. (2007). Work trajectories, income changes, and food insufficiency in a Michigan welfare population. *Social Service Review, 81*, 3–25.

Institute of Medicine. (2002). *Dietary reference intakes for energy, carbohydrate, fiber, fat, fatty acids, cholesterol, protein, and amino acids.* Washington, DC: National Academy Press.

Kim, M., Ohls, J., & Cohen, R. (2001). *Hunger in America 2001: National report prepared for America's Second Harvest.* Princeton, NJ: Mathematica Policy Research.

Laraia, B., Siega-Riz, A. Gundersen, C., & Dole, N. (2006). Psychosocial factors and socioeconomic indicators are associated with household food insecurity among pregnant women. *Journal of Nutrition, 136*, 177–182.

Lee, J., & Frongillo, E., Jr. (2001). Factors associated with food insecurity among US elderly persons: Importance of functional impairments. *Journal of Gerontology, 56B*, 594–599.

Martin, K., Rogers, B., Cook, J., & Joseph, H. (2004). Social capital is associated with decreased risk of hunger. *Social Science and Medicine, 58*, 2645–2654.

Ribar, D., & Hamrick, K. (2003). *Dynamics of poverty and food sufficiency.* Economic Research Service, Food Assistance and Nutrition Research Report, 33. Washington, DC: US Department of Agriculture.

Van Hook J., & Balistreri, K. (2006). Ineligible parents, eligible children: Food stamps receipt, allotments, and food insecurity among children of immigrants. *Social Science Research, 35*(1), 228–251.

CHAPTER 8

THE CONSEQUENCES OF FOOD INSECURITY IN THE UNITED STATES

Craig Gundersen, PhD

Chapter Objectives

After reading the chapter and reflecting on the contents, you should be able to:

1. Provide an overview of outcomes of food insecurity at both the household and the individual child level.
2. Explain how food insecurity rather than other correlated factors is responsible for the differing outcomes.
3. Discuss how childhood obesity might be related to food insecurity.
4. Understand the complex nature of food insecurity on individual outcomes.

Key Terms

at risk of overweight children: Children who are between the 85th and 95th percentile for body mass index (BMI).

child food insecurity measure: A measure made up of the food insecurity questions in the Core Food Security Module that are child specific.

household food insecurity measure: A measure made up of the food insecurity questions in the Core Food Security Module that are household specific.

overweight children: Children who are in the 95th percentile or higher for body mass index (BMI).

Introduction

Chapter 7 demonstrated why some families are more likely to be food insecure than other families. Policy makers and program administrators then use this information to help direct assistance to people who are most in danger of being food insecure. The reason for this concern about food insecurity is due, in part, to the mere existence of food insecurity—we might be concerned about people going hungry in the United States due to lack of resources. Another possible reason is that we as a society are also concerned with the consequences of food insecurity. In this chapter we examine these consequences.

The first section of this chapter presents summary statistics, in a series of bar graphs, about the differences in various outcomes by food insecurity status as measured at both the household and the child level. This will give the reader some sense as to what sorts of consequences are present. The second section then reviews the evidence regarding, controlling for other factors, whether food insecurity, rather than other correlated factors, is responsible for these differences. The third and final section covers one particular outcome that has received a great deal of attention lately: whether food insecurity is positively, negatively, or unrelated to childhood obesity.

Descriptions of the Differences in Health Outcomes by Food Insecurity Status for Children in the United States

In this section a comparison of health outcomes by food insecurity status is presented for the United States. We do so in Figures 8.1–8.12, where the comparisons are made with respect to food insecurity defined for all members of the household and for just the children in the household.

For these analyses, we used data from the 1999 to 2002 National Health and Nutrition Examination Survey (NHANES). The NHANES, conducted by the National Center for Health Statistics, Centers for Disease Control (NCHS/CDC), is a program of studies designed to assess the health and nutritional status of adults and children in the United States through interviews and direct physical examinations. The survey now examines a nationally representative sample of about 5000 persons each year, about half of whom are children. The interview includes demographic, socioeconomic, dietary, and health-related questions with components consisting of medical and dental examinations, physiological measurements, and laboratory tests. We used information from the following modules: demographics, food security, occupation, health insurance, anxiety, panic disorder, depression, body measures, medical conditions, hospital utilization, and physical functioning. As noted in Chapters 6 and 7, because food insecurity is rare among households above 200% of the poverty line, we limit our sample to households with incomes below this threshold. Our sample contains 5273 children.

As seen in Figures 8.1, 8.2, and 8.3, when one looks at differences in health outcomes by food insecurity status, differences in the percentage of children with asthma, attention deficit disorder (ADD), and learning disabilities, respectively, exist. However, at both levels of food insecurity—food insecurity defined for all members of the household and for just the children in the household—the difference between children who experience food security or food insecurity is statistically insignificant.

However, when one looks at other differences in health outcomes by food insecurity status, food insecurity status is important. Figures 8.4 and 8.5 distinguish the variation in the percentage of children with an ear infection and headache respectively. Children from food

FIGURE 8.1   Percentage of Children with Asthma by Food Insecurity

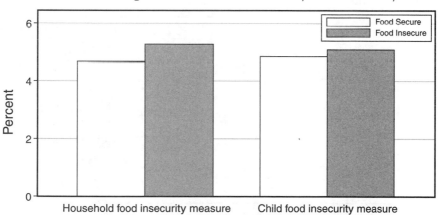

Source: Calculations by Gundersen based on data from the 1999 to 2002 National Health and Nutrition Examination Survey (NHANES).

FIGURE 8.2   Percentage of Children with ADD by Food Insecurity Status

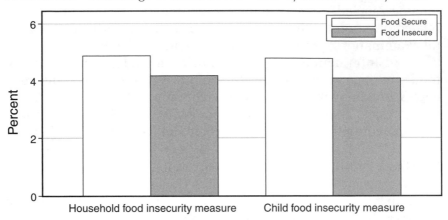

Source: Calculations by Gundersen based on data from the 1999 to 2002 National Health and Nutrition Examination Survey (NHANES).

insecure households are more likely to have an ear infection and a headache than their food secure counterparts. For example, defined over child food insecurity, Figure 8.4 shows that 8.5% of food insecure children have an ear infection versus 6.4% of food secure children. Similarly, Figure 8.5 shows that 15.4% of food insecure

FIGURE 8.3   Percentage of Children with a Learning Disability by Food Insecurity Status

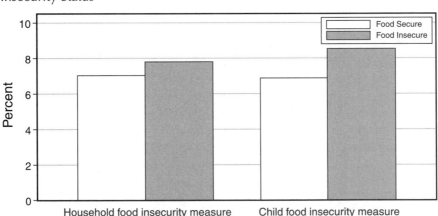

Source: Calculations by Gundersen based on data from the 1999 to 2002 National Health and Nutrition Examination Survey (NHANES).

FIGURE 8.4   Percentage of Children with an Ear Infection by Food Insecurity Status

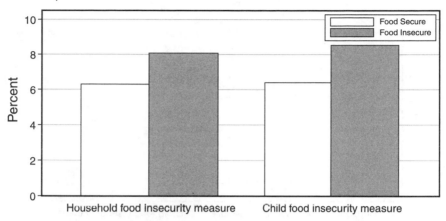

Source: Calculations by Gundersen based on data from the 1999 to 2002 National Health and Nutrition Examination Survey (NHANES).

children have a headache versus 12.5% of food secure children who have a headache.

Other child outcomes that were examined are the number of days that children miss school. Figures 8.6 and 8.7 show that food secure children are more likely to miss school for 5 or more days or for 10

FIGURE 8.5   Percentage of Children with a Headache by Food Insecurity Status

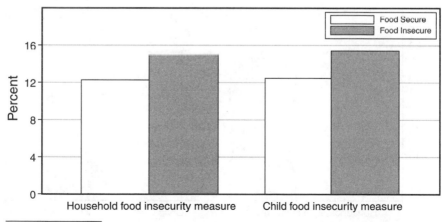

Source: Calculations by Gundersen based on data from the 1999 to 2002 National Health and Nutrition Examination Survey (NHANES).

FIGURE 8.6   Percentage of Children Missing Five or More Days of School by Food Insecurity Status

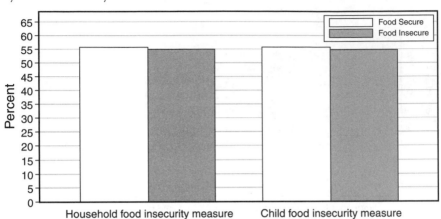

Source: Calculations by Gundersen based on data from the 1999 to 2002 National Health and Nutrition Examination Survey (NHANES).

or more days. The gap is wider when defined over child food insecurity. For example, 48.6% of food secure children miss 10 or more days of school versus 41.5% of food insecure children.

   Another difference in health outcomes by food insecurity status for which children were analyzed is childhood obesity, termed as a

FIGURE 8.7   Percentage of Children Missing 10 or More Days of School by Food Insecurity Status

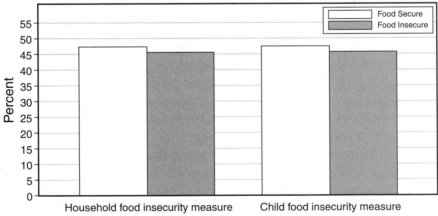

Source: Calculations by Gundersen based on data from the 1999 to 2002 National Health and Nutrition Examination Survey (NHANES).

child being in the 95th percentile or higher for body mass index (BMI). As seen in Figure 8.8, when defined over household food insecurity, 39.8% of food secure children are overweight versus 36.1% of food insecure children. Similarly, when defined over child food insecurity, 39.7% of food secure children are overweight versus 34.8% of food insecure children. However, Figure 8.9 shows less disparity

FIGURE 8.8   Percentage of Overweight Children by Food Insecurity Status

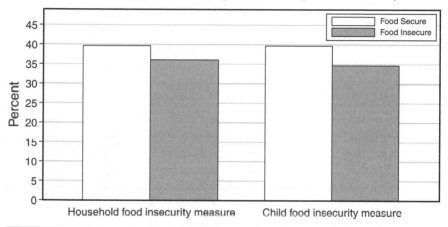

Source: Calculations by Gundersen based on data from the 1999 to 2002 National Health and Nutrition Examination Survey (NHANES).

FIGURE 8.9   Percentage of At Risk of Overweight or Overweight Children by Food Insecurity Status

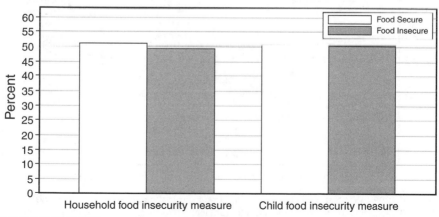

Source: Calculations by Gundersen based on data from the 1999 to 2002 National Health and Nutrition Examination Survey (NHANES).

between food secure children and food insecure children when the category of at risk of overweight is included with being overweight, termed as a child being in the 85th percentile or higher for BMI.

As seen in Figures 8.10, 8.11, and 8.12, food insecure children have worse overall health. When defined over child food insecurity,

FIGURE 8.10   Percentage of Children in Excellent Health by Food Insecurity Status

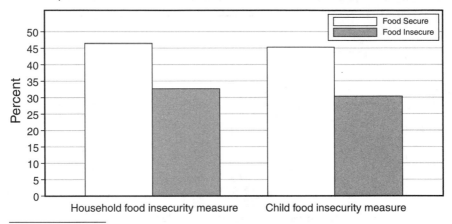

Source: Calculations by Gundersen based on data from the 1999 to 2002 National Health and Nutrition Examination Survey (NHANES).

FIGURE 8.11   Percentage of Children in Excellent or Very Good Health by Food Insecurity Status

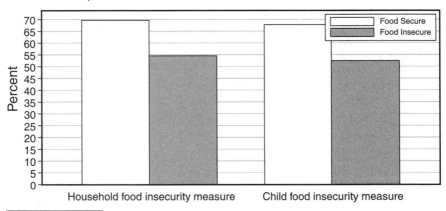

Source: 1999–2002 National Health and Nutrition Examination Survey (NHANES). The NHANES, conducted by the National Center for Health Statistics, Centers for Disease Control (NCHS/CDC).

FIGURE 8.12   Percentage of Children in Excellent, Very Good, or Good Health by Food Insecurity Status

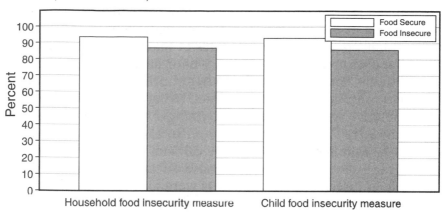

Source: Calculations by Gundersen based on data from the 1999 to 2002 National Health and Nutrition Examination Survey (NHANES).

Figure 8.10 shows that 45.2% of food secure children have excellent health versus 30.4% of food insecure children. Similarly, Figure 8.11 shows that 68% of food secure children are in excellent or very good health versus 52.5% of food insecure children. In addition, Figure 8.12 shows that only 7% of food secure children are in poor health versus 14.3% of food insecure children.

Studies of the Consequences of Food Insecurity in the United States

We now turn to a series of papers that have analyzed the consequences of food insecurity in the United States. These papers have appeared in a wide variety of journals across a wide variety of disciplines. Moreover, they use many different statistical techniques and data sets to ascertain the effect of food insecurity and other factors on health outcomes.

Dietary Intakes by Food Insecurity Status

Dixon, Winkleby, and Radimer (2001) examined whether dietary intakes and serum nutrients differed between adults from food secure

from the Fragile Families and Child Wellbeing Study, an ongoing birth-cohort study. Between 2001 and 2003, a group of 2870 mothers of 3-year-olds from 18 cities were surveyed after birth and approximately 1 and 3 years after delivery. Logistic-regression models were used to determine if the level of food insecurity increased the chances of depression or anxiety among mothers and the chances of behavior problems among their children.

After controlling for sociodemographic factors as well as maternal health, alcohol and drug use, prenatal smoking, and physical domestic violence, results showed that the percentage of mothers with depression or anxiety increased as the level of food insecurity increased: from 16.9% for food secure mothers to 21.0% for marginally food secure mothers to 30.3% for food insecure mothers. Similarly, after further controlling for maternal depression and anxiety, the percentage of children with a behavior problem increased as the level of food insecurity increased: from 22.7% for food secure children to 31.1% for marginally food secure children to 36.7% for food insecure children.

Food Insecurity and Child Behaviors

Using data from the first and second waves of the Illinois Families Study (IFS), Slack and Yoo (2005) examined the links between food insecurity and child behavior problems using hierarchical regression analyses for two different groups of children (3–5 years and 6–12 years). After controlling for parental characteristics including stress, warmth, and depression, food insecurity was determined to have an indirect association with behavior problems. Among the young children, food insecurity is mediated by parental characteristics with both externalizing and internalizing problems. However, among the older children, food insecurity is positively and indirectly associated with internalizing behavior problems by parental characteristics.

Is There a Relationship between Food Insecurity and Childhood Obesity?

Along with food insecurity, another important public health concern is childhood obesity. This current epidemic of pediatric obesity in the United States has been well documented (Ogden et al., 2006;

Koplan, Liverman, & Kraak, 2005). Recent estimates indicate that 17.1% of US children and adolescents between the ages of 2 and 19 are considered to be overweight, and another 16.5% are considered to be at risk of overweight (Ogden et al., 2006). Overweight youths have an increased likelihood of numerous medical conditions, such as elevated blood pressure and cholesterol, insulin resistance, and psychosocial disorders (Daniels, 2006). Pediatric obesity has generally been linked to energy balance, namely physical inactivity and diet (Anderson & Butcher, 2006). The latter construct is most often considered in the context of excess total energy intake (kJ/d) and/or inadequate composition (e.g., dietary fat, fruit and vegetables, etc.). (The discussion in this section borrows heavily from Gundersen et al., 2008.)

Early studies of poverty and child growth clearly show compromised growth and underweight (Tanner, 1962); hence, it is somewhat counterintuitive that food insecure children would be overweight. Consistent with this notion, some studies have found either no relationship (Alaimo, Olson, & Frongillo, 2001; Kaiser et al., 2002; Martin & Ferris, 2007) or an inverse relationship (Jimenez-Cruz, Bacardi-Gascon, & Spindler, 2003; Rose & Bodor, 2006; Matheson, Varady, Varady, & Killen, 2002) between food insecurity and child obesity. However, recent studies (Dubois, Farmer, Girard, & Porcherie, 2006; Casey, Szeto, Lensing, Bogle, & Weber, 2001; Jyoti, Frongillo, & Jones, 2005; Casey et al., 2006) have provided some evidence for a positive link between food insecurity and overweight among children.

One important methodological issue of these previous studies is that food insecurity was measured at the household level, either defined for all household members or for all children in the household. Except in cases where there is only one child in a household, the structure of the CFSM food insecurity questions does not allow for the identification of the food insecurity status of an individual child in the household. As a consequence, studies using the CFSM have not directly connected the food insecurity status of an individual child in the household with his or her own weight status.

In contrast, in Gundersen et al. (2008), the relationship between food insecurity and overweight was measured directly. Instead of defining food insecurity at the household level or for all children in the household, the authors examined the association between food insecurity and overweight status when food insecurity and BMI are measured for the same child. They did so with data from the first wave of Welfare, Children, and Families: A Three-City Study (commonly referred to as the Three-City Study), which focuses on the well-being of low-income children and families. These data provide in-depth information for focal children in these families, including food insecurity and weight status.

Their study found that food insecurity was not associated with an increased or decreased risk of overweight in low-income children when food insecurity and BMI are measured for the same focal child. In other words, food insecure children were no more likely than food secure children to be overweight or at risk of overweight. This is consistent with the work of Alaimo et al. (2001), Kaiser et al. (2002), and Martin and Ferris (2007). There are at least three possible reasons for the findings in Gundersen et al. (2008). First, previous studies that used household measures of food insecurity might have masked differences between individuals within a household. By examining just a single child, one can isolate the more direct impact of food insecurity on obesity. Second, along with masking differences between individuals, the standard household-based food insecurity module used in previous research is designed to portray both worries about reductions in food intakes and actual intake reductions. In contrast, the measures of individual (i.e., focal child) food insecurity used in Gundersen et al. consider reductions in food intake without reference to worries. As a result, standard household food security measures might be capturing something distinct from food security assessments at the individual level. For example, worries about reductions in food intake might be associated with stress, and stress has been associated with obesity (Bjorntorp, 2001). It is plausible that the stress evident within the household is behind the positive relation between food insecurity and obesity found in previous studies. Third, as noted above, the questions in their study were drawn from the child-specific questions in the CFSM and assess relatively more severe levels of food insecurity (Gundersen et al., 2008). Thus, it might be that the less severe levels of food insecurity examined in earlier studies are associated with obesity, while the more severe levels portrayed in Gundersen et al. are not associated with obesity.

While food insecure children were no more likely than food secure children to be overweight or at risk of overweight in their study, an important point (and paradox) still remains—that is, food insecurity and overweight coexist in low-income children. In their sample, one-fourth of food insecure children were overweight, and almost half were at risk of overweight or overweight. The possible reasons for this paradox might include overconsumption of cheaper, energy-dense foods (Dietz, 1995; Drewnowski & Specter, 2004), overeating in times when food is more plentiful (Scheier, 2005), metabolic changes to ensure a more efficient use of energy (Alaimo et al., 2001), different standards of what constitutes an adequate diet (Gundersen & Ribar, 2005), parents overprotecting their children by giving them more food than needed when food is available (McIntyre et al., 2003), and the mother being food insecure during pregnancy (Laraia, Siega-Riz, Gundersen, & Dole, 2006).

Chapter Summary

As a society, we are concerned about food insecurity and its consequences. Several studies have been undertaken to examine the consequences of food insecurity. In addition to our basic concern of people going hungry, research has shown that several other consequences are associated with higher levels of food insecurity. After controlling for other factors, mediators of food insecurity have been found, which allow food insecurity to indirectly have an influence on several key health outcomes.

Issues to Debate

1. Discuss examples of food insecurity indirectly influencing negative child outcomes focusing on how these outcomes might affect the child's future.
2. Discuss what sorts of policies the United States might want to pursue to alleviate food insecurity based on the consequences and outcomes learned thus far.

References

Alaimo, K., Olson, C. M., & Frongillo, E. A. (2001). Low family income and food insufficiency in relation to overweight in US children: Is there a paradox? *Archives of Pediatric and Adolescent Medicine, 155,* 1161–1167.

Anderson, P. M., & Butcher, K. E. (2006). Childhood obesity: Trends and potential causes. *Future Child, 16*, 19–45.

Bjorntorp, P. (2001). Do stress reactions cause abdominal obesity and comorbidities? *Obesity Reviews, 2*, 73–86.

Bronte-Tinkew, J., Zaslow, M., Capps, R., Horowitz, A., & McNamara, M. (2007). Food insecurity works through depression, parenting, and infant feeding to influence overweight and health in toddlers. *Journal of Nutrition, 137*, 2160–2165.

Carmichael, S. L., Yang, W., Herring, A., Abrams, B., & Shaw, G. M. (2007). Maternal food insecurity is associated with increased risk of certain birth defects. *Journal of Nutrition, 137*, 2087–2092.

Casey, P., Simpson, P., Gossett, J., Bogle, M., Champagne, C., Connell, C., et al. (2006). The association of child and household food insecurity with childhood overweight status. *Pediatrics, 118*, 1406–1413.

Casey, P., Szeto, K., Lensing, S., Bogle, M., & Weber, J. (2001). Children in food-insufficient, low-income families: Prevalence, health and nutrition status. *Archives of Pediatric and Adolescent Medicine, 155*, 508–514.

Daniels, S. R. (2006). The consequences of childhood overweight and obesity. *Future Child, 16*, 47–67.

Dietz, W. H. (1995). Does hunger cause obesity? *Pediatrics, 95*, 766–767.

Dixon, L. B., Winkleby, M. A., & Radimer, K. L. (2001). Dietary intakes and serum nutrients differ between adults from food-insufficient and food-sufficient families: Third national health and nutrition examination survey, 1988–1994. *Journal of Nutrition, 131*, 1232–1246.

Drewnowski, A., & Specter, S. E. (2004). Poverty and obesity: The role of energy density and energy costs. *American Journal of Clinical Nutrition, 79*, 6–16.

Dubois, L., Farmer, A., Girard, M., & Porcherie, M. (2006). Family food insufficiency is related to overweight among preschoolers. *Social Science and Medicine, 63*, 1503–1516.

Gundersen, C., Lohman, B., Eisenmann, J., Garasky, S., & Stewart, S. (2008). Lack of association between child-specific food insecurity and overweight in a sample of 10–15 year old low-income youth. *Journal of Nutrition, 138*, 371–378.

Gundersen, C., & Ribar, D. (2005). *Food insecurity and insufficiency at low levels of food expenditures* (Working Paper No. 1594). Institute for the Study of Labor (IZA).

Jimenez-Cruz, A., Bacardi-Gascon, M., & Spindler, A. (2003). Obesity and hunger among Mexican-Indian migrant children on the US–Mexico border. *International Journal of Obesity, 27*, 740–747.

Jyoti, D. F., Frongillo, E. A., & Jones, S. J. (2005). Food insecurity affects school children's academic performance, weight gain, and social skills. *Journal of Nutrition, 135*, 2831–2839.

Kaiser, L., Melgar-Quiñonez, H., Lamp, C., Johns, M., Sutherlin, J., & Harwood, J. (2002). Food security and nutritional outcomes of preschool-age Mexican-American children. *Journal of the American Dietetic Association, 102*, 924–929.

Koplan, J., Liverman, C., & Kraak, V. (Eds.). (2005). *Preventing childhood obesity: Health in the balance*. Washington, DC: National Academies Press.

Laraia, B., Siega-Riz, A., Gundersen, C., & Dole, N. (2006). Psychosocial factors and socioeconomic indicators are associated with household food insecurity among pregnant women. *Journal of Nutrition, 136,* 177–182.

Martin, K. S., & Ferris, A. M. (2007). Food insecurity and gender are risk factors for obesity. *Journal of Nutrition Education and Behavior, 39,* 31–36.

Matheson, D., Varady, J., Varady, A., & Killen, J. (2002). Household food security and nutritional status of Hispanic children in the fifth grade. *American Journal of Clinical Nutrition, 76,* 210–217.

McIntyre, L., Glanville, N., Raine, K., Dayle, J., Anderson, B., & Battaglia, N. (2003). Do low-income lone mothers compromise their nutrition to feed their children? *Canadian Medical Association Journal, 198,* 686–691.

Ogden, C. L., Carroll, M. D., Curtin, L. R., McDowell, M. A., Tabak, C. J., & Flegal, K. M. (2006). Prevalence of overweight and obesity in the United States, 1999–2004. *Journal of the American Medical Association, 295,* 1549–1555.

Rose, D., & Bodor, J. (2006). Household food insecurity and overweight status in young school children: Results from the early childhood longitudinal study. *Pediatrics, 117,* 464–473.

Scheier, L. M. (2005). What is the hunger–obesity paradox. *Journal of the American Dietetic Association, 105,* 883–886.

Slack, K., & Yoo, J. (2005). Food hardship and child behavior problems among low-income children. *Social Service Review, 75,* 511–536.

Tanner, J. M. (1962). *Growth at adolescence* (2nd ed.). Oxford, England: Blackwell Press.

Whitaker, R. C., Phillips, S. M., & Orzol, S. M. (2006). Food insecurity and the risks of depression and anxiety in mothers and behavior problems in their pre-school-aged children. *Pediatrics, 118,* e859–e868.

CHAPTER 9

FOOD ASSISTANCE PROGRAMS IN THE UNITED STATES

Craig Gundersen, PhD

Chapter Objectives

After reading the chapter and reflecting on the contents, you should be able to:

1. Provide an overview of five federal food programs designed to alleviate food insecurity.
2. Compare and contrast these federal food programs.
3. Discuss which types of low-income individuals are eligible for benefits.
4. Understand how the federal food programs offer nutrition education in addition to food benefits and how this can affect the health of the programs' recipients.

Key Terms

Food Stamp Program (FSP): A federal program that helps needy persons to obtain a low-cost, nutritionally adequate diet by increasing their food purchasing ability.

National School Breakfast Program (NSBP): A federally assisted meal program that operates in public and nonprofit private schools and residential child care institutions and assists schools with serving breakfasts to needy children.

National School Lunch Program (NSLP): A federally assisted meal program that operates in public and nonprofit private schools and residential child care institutions and provides nutritionally balanced, low-cost or free lunches to children each school day.

Special Supplemental Nutrition Program for Women, Infants, and Children (WIC): A federal grant program that targets low-income, nutritionally at-risk pregnant, postpartum, and breast-feeding women and infants and children up to age 5 by providing nutritious foods, nutrition education, and referrals to health and other social services at no charge.

The Emergency Food Assistance Program (TEFAP): A federal program that supplements the diets of low-income people by providing them with emergency food assistance.

Introduction

Chapters 6, 7, and 8 covered how food insecurity is defined, an overview of food insecurity in the United States, the determinants of food insecurity, and the consequences of food insecurity. In response to the problems associated with food insecurity and, more broadly, the nutrition-related challenges facing low-income families, the US government has implemented a series of food assistance programs. In this chapter we examine these programs.

We begin with a discussion of the largest food assistance program in the United States, the Food Stamp Program. We then turn to three programs directed toward children in the United States: the Special Supplemental Nutrition Program for Women, Infants, and Children (WIC); the National School Lunch Program; and the National School Breakfast Program. We conclude with a discussion of The Emergency Food Assistance Program (TEFAP).

Food Stamp Program

The Food Stamp Program is by far the largest US food assistance program, serving approximately 26.7 million individuals in 2006 with an annual benefit distribution of $32.9 billion (Wolkwitz, 2007). Participants receive benefits for the purchase of food in authorized, privately run retail food outlets that sell food to participants and nonparticipants. Benefits are distributed via an Electronic Benefit Transfer (EBT) card, which is operationally similar to an ATM card. These benefits are inversely related to income. The central goal of the

Food Stamp Program is to be a core component of the safety net against hunger (US Department of Agriculture, 1999, p. 7).

History

The Food Stamp Program (FSP) has a long history filled with many modifications. The Food Stamp Program began in a very early form in 1939 when needy people were allowed to buy orange stamps equal to their normal food expenditures and then receive supplemental blue stamps that were valued at 50% of the household's normal food expenditures. Although orange stamps could be used to buy any food, blue stamps could only be used to buy food that the US Department of Agriculture (USDA) determined to be surplus. In 1961, a new pilot Food Stamp Program was initiated that retained the requirement that the food stamps be purchased but eliminated stamps specifically for surplus foods. On August 31, 1964, the Food Stamp Act of 1964 was passed with the following major provisions: (1) each state developed the eligibility standards to use within its borders; (2) recipients purchased their food stamps, paying an amount corresponding with their normal food expenditures and then received a predetermined amount of food stamps based on the income needed to obtain a low-cost, nutritionally adequate diet; (3) all food items except alcoholic beverages and imported foods were deemed suitable for purchase with food stamps; (4) discrimination on the basis of race, religious creed, national origin, or political beliefs was prohibited; and (5) the division of responsibilities between the states and the federal government were outlined.

By the 1970s, changes were needed to keep up with increased rates of participation. The Food Stamp Act of 1977 made a major change by eliminating the so-called purchase requirement. Under this purchase requirement, recipients had to pay for the food stamps on a sliding scale proportional to their income. In other words, as a household's income rose, participants had to pay more for food stamps. This purchase requirement was thought to discourage participation. Consistent with this, with the elimination of the purchase requirement on January 1, 1979, there was a 1.5 million participant increase that month over the preceding month. By the mid- to late-1980s, domestic hunger was recognized as a severe problem in the United States and led to further improvements in the FSP, such as elimination of sales taxes on food stamp purchases, the reinstatement of categorical eligibility, an increased resource limit, eligibility for homeless persons, and expansion of nutrition education.

More recently, several changes to the Food Stamp Program occurred. The 1993 Mickey Leland Childhood Hunger Relief Act included changes that allowed households with children to more easily gain access to needed food stamp benefits. Changes included raising the cap on the dependent care deduction and simplifying the household definition. The Personal Responsibility and Work Opportunities Reconciliation Act of 1996 (PRWORA) enacted other major changes to the FSP including: (1) restricting the eligibility of most legal immigrants to food stamps, (2) placing a time limit on food stamp receipt for healthy adults with no dependent children, and (3) requiring states to implement the EBT system.

Finally, in May 2002, the Food Security and Rural Investment Act of 2002 included further changes to food stamps, including: (1) the reestablishment of eligibility to qualified legal immigrants, (2) the modification of the standard deduction to vary by household size and to adjust each year for inflation, (3) the use of a common definition of income and/or benefits in federal programs, and (4) the provision of incentives to encourage states to maintain high standards within the administration of the program. In addition, the 2002 Farm Bill restored food stamp eligibility to most legal immigrants. Legal immigrants may be eligible for the food stamp benefits that meet the following additional requirements: (1) have lived in the country for 5 years; (2) are receiving disability-related assistance or benefits, regardless of entry date; or (3) are children regardless of entry date. Certain noncitizens, such as those admitted for humanitarian reasons, are also eligible for food stamp benefits. Eligible household members can get food stamps even if other members of the household are not eligible. However, noncitizens that are in the United States temporarily, such as students, are not eligible.

Eligibility Criteria

To first define who is eligible, the relevant unit is established. For food stamps, this is defined at the household. More specifically, a household is defined as one containing people who live together and purchase and prepare meals together. However, if a person is 60 years of age or older and unable to purchase and prepare meals separately because of a permanent disability, the person, and the person's spouse if applicable, may be a separate household if those with whom he or she lives are considered to be low income.

To be eligible for food stamps, households have to first meet a monthly gross income test. Under this criterion, a household's income (before any deductions) has to be less than 130% of the poverty line. As an example, in 2008, a food stamp household with three persons and a monthly income less than $1861 would be gross income eligible. The gross income test does not apply to all households, however; households with at least one elderly member or one disabled member do not have to meet this test.

Households with an elderly or disabled member and most all other households have to pass the net income criteria as well, where net income is defined as gross income minus certain deductions. The allowable deductions include: (1) a standard deduction for all households; (2) a 20% earned income deduction; (3) a dependent care deduction when care is necessary for work, training, or education; (4) a legally owed child support payments deduction; (5) a medical costs deduction for elderly and disabled people; and (6) an excess shelter cost deduction. To be eligible, this net income must be less than the poverty line. As an example, in 2008, a food stamp household with net income below $1431 would be net income eligible. Households in which all members receive SSI or TANF benefits are considered to be automatically eligible for food stamps and do not have to pass either the gross or the net income tests.

The final test for food stamp eligibility is the asset test. For most households, the total assets of a household must be under $2000. When determining eligibility with respect to assets, some resources are not counted, such as one's home and up to $4650 of the fair market value of one car per adult household member. Similarly, one car per teenaged household member may be deducted if the teenager is using it for work, and a vehicle's value is not counted if it is needed to transport a physically disabled household member.

Two exceptions to these rules apply. First, households with an elderly or disabled person have a higher asset limit: $3000. Second, households where everyone receives SSI or TANF benefits are not subject to the asset test.

In general, there are not work requirements for food stamp recipients. However, able-bodied adults between the ages of 18 and 50 years must be employed to receive food stamps. If they are not employed, they can lose their food stamp benefits. In areas with particularly high unemployment rates or limited employment opportunities, this so-called "ABAWD requirement" is waived.

Nonparticipation by Eligible Persons

A high proportion of households that are eligible for food stamps do not participate. This outcome is often ascribed to three main factors. First, there can be stigma associated with receiving food stamps. Stigma encompasses a wide variety of sources, from a person's own distaste for receiving food stamps to the fear of disapproval from others when redeeming food stamps to the possible negative reaction of caseworkers (Ranney & Kushman, 1987; Moffitt, 1983). Second, transaction costs can diminish the attractiveness of participation. Examples of such costs include travel time to a food stamp office and time spent in the office, the burden of transporting children to the office or paying for child care services, and the direct costs of paying for transportation. A household faces these costs on a repeated basis when it must recertify its eligibility. Third, the benefit level can be quite small—for some families as low as $10 per month.

Because the Government Performance and Results Act of 1993 calls for policy makers to assess the effects of federal programs, the extent of nonparticipation by eligible households is closely followed. To this end, the national food stamp participation rate, defined as the percentage of eligible people who actually participate in food stamps, has been used to assess performance for nearly 25 years. In 2008, a performance target of 68% of the eligible population was set to be reached by 2010.

The most recently calculated food stamp participation rates show that about 65% of eligible people in the United States received food stamp benefits in 2005. However, participation rates varied greatly from state to state. Missouri, Tennessee, Oregon, Maine, West Virginia, Oklahoma, Louisiana, and Kentucky had significantly higher participation rates than two-thirds of the remaining states, while Wyoming, Nevada, California, and Massachusetts had significantly lower rates. Furthermore, in 2005, among the eligible working poor—those who work but are still in need—57% received food stamps. Similar to the participation rates for all eligible people, rates for the working poor varied widely across states.

The Special Supplemental Nutrition Program for Women, Infants, and Children (WIC)

The goal of the Special Supplemental Nutrition Program for Women, Infants, and Children (WIC) in the United States' social safety net is to "provide supplemental nutritious food as an adjunct to good health during such critical times of growth and development [during pregnancy, the postpartum period, infancy, and early childhood] in order to prevent the occurrence of health problems" (P.L. 94–105). To meet this goal, WIC provides nutritious foods, nutrition education, and referrals to health and other social services to participants. WIC targets low-income, nutritionally at-risk pregnant, postpartum, and breast-feeding women, and infants and children up to age 5 years. WIC is not an entitlement program, meaning that Congress does not set aside funds to allow every eligible individual to participate in the program. Instead, WIC is a federal grant program for which Congress authorizes a specific amount of funding each year. The USDA, through its Food and Nutrition Service, provides these funds to WIC state agencies, such as state health departments, to pay for WIC foods, nutrition education, and administrative costs. WIC operates through 2000 local agencies in 10,000 clinic sites, in 50 state health departments, 34 Indian Tribal Organizations, the District of Columbia, and five territories (Northern Mariana, American Samoa, Guam, Puerto Rico, and the Virgin Islands).

History

WIC was launched as a pilot program in 1972 and made permanent in 1974. Formerly known as the Special Supplemental Food Program for Women, Infants, and Children, WIC's name was changed to emphasize its role as a nutrition program under the Healthy Meals for Healthy Americans Act of 1994. Most state WIC programs provide food vouchers that participants use at authorized stores. A wide variety of state and local organizations collaborate in providing the food and health care benefits with over 45,000 merchants nationally accepting WIC vouchers.

Participation in WIC has slowly but steadily grown over the years. In 1974, 88,000 people participated. By 1980, participation was at 1.9 million. By 1990, participation more than doubled to 4.5

million. By 2004, the average monthly participation was approximately 7.9 million. Of the 7.9 million people who received WIC benefits, approximately 4 million were children, 2 million were infants, and 1.9 million were women. Currently, WIC serves 45% of all infants (up to the first birthday) who are born in the United States.

In 2007, the projected total costs for WIC were $5.4 billion, with $3.9 billion covering food costs and the remainder covering nutrition service and administrative costs. By comparison, the WIC program appropriation was $21 million in 1974 and increased to $750 million by 1980.

Eligibility Criteria

Eligibility for the WIC program is at the individual level. Pregnant or postpartum women, infants, and children up to age 5 years are eligible. They must meet income guidelines, a state residency requirement, and be individually determined to be at "nutrition risk" by a health professional. To be eligible on the basis of income, an applicant's income must fall at or below 185% of the poverty threshold, which is $38,203 in 2008 for a family of four. A person who participates or has family members who participate in other selected benefit programs (e.g., the Food Stamp Program) automatically meets the income eligibility requirement.

In addition to the income requirement, an individual must be nutritionally at risk. To be determined to be at nutrition risk, two major types of nutrition risk are recognized for WIC eligibility. The first type of risk includes medically based risks such as anemia, underweight, overweight, history of pregnancy complications, or poor pregnancy outcomes. The second type of risk includes dietary risks, such as failure to meet the dietary guidelines or inappropriate nutrition practices. This health screening is free to program applicants.

Because WIC cannot serve all eligible people, a system of priorities has been established for filling program openings. When a local WIC agency has reached its maximum caseload, vacancies are filled based on this system of priority levels. The highest priority is given to pregnant women, breast-feeding women, and infants who are determined to be at nutrition risk because of a nutrition-related medical condition. The second highest priority level consists of infants up to 6 months of age whose mothers participated in WIC or could have participated and had a serious medical problem. Children at nutrition risk because of a nutrition-related medical problem are third on this priority list. The next in priority are pregnant or breast-feeding women and infants at nutrition risk because of an inadequate dietary pattern, followed by children at nutrition risk because of an inadequate dietary pattern. The sixth priority level is reserved for nonbreast-feeding, postpartum women with any nutrition risk. The final level in this priority level system consists of individuals at nutrition risk only because they are homeless or migrants, and current participants who, without WIC foods, could continue to have medical and/or dietary problems.

Research on the Benefits of WIC

WIC has become a very popular program among policy makers in the United States. The reasons for this are due, in part, to the demonstrated success of WIC. For example, previous research has demonstrated that WIC is an important service program insofar as, in comparison to eligible nonparticipants, WIC recipients have fewer small-for-gestational-age births (Ahluwalia, Hogan, Grummer-Strawn, Colville, & Peterson, 1998; Brown, Watkins, & Hiett, 1996), have lower infant mortality rates (Moss & Carver, 1998), have higher birth weights (Devaney, Bilheimer, & Schore, 1992; Kowaleski-Jones & Duncan, 2002), purchase more nutritious foods (Arcia, Crouch, & Kulka, 1990), have higher nutrient intakes (Oliveira & Gundersen, 2000), have lower levels of maternal anemia (Kim, Hungerford, Kuester, Zyrkowski, & Trowbridge, 1992; Yip et al., 1992), are healthier (Carlson & Senauer, 2003), and have better birth outcomes across a wide variety of measures (Bitler & Currie, 2005).

National School Lunch Program

The National School Lunch Program (NSLP) is a federally assisted meal program that operates in over 101,000 public and nonprofit private schools and residential child care institutions. It provides nutritionally balanced, low-cost, or free lunches to children each school day. In 2007, over 30 million students participated in NSLP. Of these students, nearly 15 million received free lunches, while 3 million received reduced-price lunches. In addition, over 12 million students paid full price at schools that receive federal subsidies. Of the total number of school lunches served in 2007, almost three in five were free or reduced-price lunches. In addition to any commodities the schools received, the cash payments to schools for the NSLP in 2007 were almost $8 billion.

History

The program was established in 1946 under the National School Lunch Act. In 1998, Congress expanded the NSLP to include reimbursement for snacks served to all children in after-school educational and enrichment programs. At the federal level, the USDA, through its Food and Nutrition Service, administers the program. At the state level, the NSLP is usually administered by state education agencies that operate the program through agreements with local school food authorities.

Eligibility Criteria

Generally, public or nonprofit private schools and residential child care institutions may participate in the NSLP. School districts and independent schools that choose to participate in the lunch program get cash subsidies and donated commodities from the USDA for each meal they serve. In return, they must serve lunches that meet federal requirements, providing no more than 30% of an individual's calories from fat, less than 10% from saturated fat, and one-third of the Recommended Dietary Allowances of protein, vitamin A, vitamin C, iron, calcium, and calories. School districts must offer free or reduced price lunches to eligible children. In addition, school food authorities can also be reimbursed for snacks served to children through age 18 years in after-school educational or enrichment programs.

Eligibility for the NSLP begins at the individual level. Any child at a participating school may purchase a meal through the NSLP. Children from families with incomes at or below 130% of the poverty level are eligible for free meals. Those children whose household income is between 130% and 185% of the poverty level are eligible for reduced-price meals, which cannot cost more than 40 cents. (In 2008, 130% of the poverty level is $26,845 for a family of four, while 185% is $38,203.) Although children from families with incomes over 185% of poverty pay a full price, their meals are still subsidized to some extent. Although local school food authorities set their own prices for full-price meals, they must operate their meal services as nonprofit programs. In addition, after-school snacks are provided to children on the same income eligibility basis as school meals. However, schools where at least 50% of students are eligible for free or reduced-price meals may receive reimbursements for all their snacks.

National School Breakfast Program

The National School Breakfast Program (NSBP) is a federally assisted meal program that operates in public and nonprofit private schools and residential child care institutions. In 2007, more than 10.1 million children participated. Of these children, more than four in five received their breakfasts free or at a reduced price. For 2007, the budget of the NSBP was more than $2 billion.

History

The NSBP began as a pilot project in 1966 to assist schools that served breakfasts to needy children who had to travel a great distance to school or who attended schools located in poor areas. The pilot program was extended several times during the next few years, resulting in a number of modifications to expand the program. In 1971, Congress included as a priority those schools in which there was a need to improve the nutrition and dietary practices of children of working mothers and children from low-income families. An even more important change occurred in 1973 when the categorical grant reimbursement system was replaced by a system of specific per-meal reimbursement. In 1975 the NSBP became a permanent federally assisted meal program. As part of the legislation making the NSBP permanent, Congress affirmed its objective that the program be available in all schools where it is needed to provide adequate nutrition for the attending children. Moreover, the legislation continued to promote participation by schools in severe need by providing them with higher reimbursements.

Participation in NSBP has grown over the years. In 1970, around 500,000 children participated, and by 1975, the number of participants had increased to 1.8 million children. By 1980, the number of participating children was 3.6 million. Twenty years later, the number of participants was more than 7.5 million children.

Eligibility Criteria

The NSBP is administered at the federal level by the USDA through its Food and Nutrition Service. At the individual state level, the program is usually administered by its education agencies, which operate the program through agreements with local school food authorities in nearly 84,000 schools and institutions. Generally, any public or nonprofit private schools and residential child care institutions can participate in the NSBP. School districts and independent schools that choose to participate in the breakfast program receive cash subsidies from the USDA for each meal they serve. In return, they must serve breakfasts that meet federal requirements, including providing no more than 30% of an individual's calories from fat, less than 10% from saturated fat, and one-fourth of the Recommended Dietary Allowance for protein, calcium, iron, vitamin A, vitamin C, and calories. In addition, they must offer free or reduced-price breakfasts to eligible children.

Participation in the NSBP requires eligibility at both the individual and school level. First, at the individual level, any child at a participating school can purchase a meal through the NSBP. To be eligible for free meals, a child's family's income must be at or below 130% of the federal poverty level. Children who families' incomes are between 130% and 185% of the poverty level are eligible for reduced-price meals. (Currently, 130% of the poverty level is $26,845 for a family of four, while 185% is $38,203.) Although children from families over 185% of poverty pay full price, their meals are still subsidized to some extent.

At the school level, schools can qualify for higher reimbursements if a specified percentage of their lunches are served free or at a reduced price. These severe need payments are up to 24 cents higher than the normal reimbursements for free and reduced-price breakfasts. About 65% of the breakfasts served in the NSBP receive severe need payments. In addition, schools can charge no more than 30 cents for a reduced-price breakfast. Although schools set their own prices for breakfasts served to students who pay the full meal price, they must operate their meal services as nonprofit programs to participate. In addition, the USDA uses Team Nutrition to provide schools with the following: (1) technical training and assistance to help school food service staffs prepare healthy meals, and (2) nutrition education to facilitate children's understanding of the connection between diet and health.

The Emergency Food Assistance Program (TEFAP)

The Emergency Food Assistance Program (TEFAP) is a federal program that supplements the diets of low-income people by providing them with emergency food assistance. In 2007, almost $200 million was allocated to TEFAP.

History

TEFAP was first authorized as the Temporary Emergency Food Assistance Program in 1981 to distribute surplus commodity foods to households. Under the 1990 Farm Bill, the name was changed to the Emergency Food Assistance Program. The program was intended to reduce federal food inventories and their accompanying storage costs while simultaneously assisting needy households. Because some of the food stocks previously held in surplus had been depleted by 1988, the Hunger Prevention Act of 1988 authorized funds to be appropriated for the purchase of commodity foods specifically for TEFAP. The foods acquired with these appropriated funds are in addition to any surplus commodity foods donated to TEFAP by the USDA.

Eligibility Criteria

Under TEFAP, the USDA makes commodity foods available to state distributing agencies. The amount of food that each particular state receives out of the total amount of food that is provided by the federal government is based on the number of unemployed persons and the number of people with incomes below the poverty level in that particular state. States supply the food to local agencies, usually food banks, which, in turn, distribute the food to local organizations, such as soup kitchens and food pantries that directly serve the public. States also give the commodity foods to other types of local organizations, such as community action agencies, which distribute the foods directly to needy households. These local organizations distribute the donated foods to low-income persons for household consumption or use them to prepare and serve meals in a congregate setting, such as those serving the homeless.

Eligibility for TEFAP is based on need. Participant eligibility requirements are based in conjunction with nonprofit organization requirements as well as individual household requirements including the homeless. Public or private nonprofit organizations that provide food assistance to needy persons through the distribution of commodity foods for either home use or the preparation of meals must do the following: (1) determine the household's eligibility by applying income standards for home use distribution, and/or (2) demonstrate that they serve predominately needy persons if prepared meals are provided.

Each state sets its own criteria for determining what households are eligible to receive food for home consumption. At the state's discretion, income standards can be met through household participation in other existing federal, state, or local programs for which eligibility is based on income. Because states set their own criteria, states can modify the income criteria to ensure that assistance is provided only to the most needy households. Recipients of prepared meals, however, are considered to be needy and are not subject to an income requirement. Specifically, homeless persons can receive prepared meals served in a congregate setting without submitting an application. However, if a homeless person is not served prepared meals and wants to receive TEFAP foods, state income eligibility requirements must be met.

Chapter Summary

As a society, we are concerned about food insecurity and other nutrition-related deficiencies experienced by millions of Americans. In response, a series of federal food assistance programs have been established. In this chapter, we covered the history, eligibility criteria, and other aspects of the largest of these programs, the Food Stamp Program, WIC, the National School Lunch Program, the National School Breakfast Program, and the Emergency Food Assistance Program.

Issues to Debate

1. Discuss how targeting different subgroups of the population affects the effectiveness and efficiency of the federal food programs' goal to alleviate food insecurity.
2. Discuss the differences in eligibility among the federal programs examined in this chapter and how these may or may not hinder the effectiveness of the programs.
3. Discuss the implications that the eligibility requirements might have on children of immigrants, most notably those of illegal immigrants.

Web Sites

Food Stamp Program Participation and Costs
http://www.fns.usda.gov/pd/fssummar.htm

Food Stamp Program Eligibility
http://www.fns.usda.gov/fsp/applicant_recipients/eligibility.htm

WIC at a Glance
http://www.fns.usda.gov/wic/aboutwic/wicataglance.htm

WIC's Mission
http://www.fns.usda.gov/wic/aboutwic/mission.htm

WIC Nutrition Program Facts Food and Nutrition Service
http://www.fns.usda.gov/wic/WIC-Fact-Sheet.pdf

How WIC Helps
http://www.fns.usda.gov/wic/aboutwic/howwichelps.htm

Frequently Asked Questions about WIC
http://www.fns.usda.gov/wic/FAQs/faq.htm

National School Lunch Program: Participation and Lunches Served
http://www.fns.usda.gov/pd/slsummar.htm

National School Lunch Program
http://www.fns.usda.gov/cnd/lunch/AboutLunch/NSLPFactSheet.pdf

National School Lunch Program—Program History
http://www.fns.usda.gov/cnd/lunch/AboutLunch/NSLP-Program
%20History.pdf

The School Breakfast Program
http://www.fns.usda.gov/cnd/breakfast/AboutBFast/SBPFactSheet.pdf

The School Breakfast Program—Program History
http://www.fns.usda.gov/cnd/breakfast/AboutBFast/ProgHistory.htm

School Breakfast Program Participation and Meals Served
http://www.fns.usda.gov/pd/sbsummar.htm

The Emergency Food Assistance Program
http://www.fns.usda.gov/fdd/programs/tefap/pfs-tefap.pdf

Food Distribution Programs History and Background
http://www.fns.usda.gov/fdd/aboutfd/history.htm

References

Ahluwalia, I., Hogan, V., Grummer-Strawn, L., Colville, W., & Peterson, A. (1998). The effect of WIC participation on small-for-gestational-age births: Michigan, 1992. *American Journal of Public Health, 88*(9), 1374–1377.

Arcia, G., Crouch, L., & Kulka, R. (1990). Impact of the WIC program on food expenditures. *American Journal of Agricultural Economics, 72,* 218–226.

Bitler, M., & Currie, J. (2005). Does WIC work? The effects of WIC on pregnancy and birth outcomes. *Journal of Policy Analysis and Management, 24,* 73–93.

Brown, H., Watkins, K., & Hiett, A. (1996). The impact of the women, infants and children food supplement program on birth outcomes. *American Journal of Obstetrics and Gynecology, 174,* 1279–1283.

Carlson, A., & Senauer, B. (2003). The impact of the Special Supplemental Nutrition Program for Women, Infants, and Children on child health. *American Journal of Agricultural Economics, 85*(2), 479–491.

Devaney, B., Bilheimer, L., & Schore, J. (1992). Medicaid costs and birth outcomes: The effects of prenatal WIC participation and the use of prenatal care. *Journal of Policy Analysis and Management, 11*(4), 573–592.

Kim, I., Hungerford, D., Kuester, S., Zyrkowski, C., & Trowbridge, F. (1992). Pregnancy nutrition surveillance system—United States, 1979–1990. *Morbidity and Mortality Weekly Report, 41*(SS-7), 26–42.

Kowaleski-Jones, L., & Duncan, G. (2002). Effects of participation in the WIC program on birthweight: Evidence from the national longitudinal survey of youth. *American Journal of Public Health, 92*(5), 799–804.

Moffitt, R. (1983). An economic model of welfare stigma. *American Economic Review, 73*, 1023–1035.

Moss, N., & Carver, K. (1998). The effect of WIC and Medicaid on infant mortality in the United States. *American Journal of Public Health, 88*(9), 1354–1361.

Oliveira, V., & Gundersen, C. (2000). *WIC and the nutrient intake of children* (Food Assistance and Nutrition Research Report, 5). US Department of Agriculture, Economic Research Service.

Ranney, C., & Kushman, J. (1987). Cash equivalence, welfare stigma, and food stamps. *Southern Economic Journal, 53*(4), 1011–1027.

US Department of Agriculture. (1999). *Food and Nutrition Service. Annual historical review: Fiscal year 1997.*

Wolkwitz, K. (2007). *Characteristics of food stamp households: Fiscal year 2006* (Nutrition Assistance Program Report Series, Report No. FSP-07 CHAR). Washington, DC: US Department of Agriculture.

Yip, R., Pravanta, I., Scanlon, K., Borland, E., Russell, C., & Trowbridge, F. (1992). Pediatric nutrition survcillance system—United States, 1980–1991. *Morbidity and Mortality Weekly Report, 41*(SS-7), 1–24.

SECTION THREE

FOOD AND BIOTERRORISM

CHAPTER 10

INTENTIONAL AND UNINTENTIONAL CONTAMINATION OF THE FOOD SUPPLY

Tamara M. Crutchley Bushell, PhD

Chapter Objectives

After reading the chapter and reflecting on the contents, you should be able to:

1. Identify key vulnerabilities in the agricultural and food infrastructures.
2. Discuss how these key vulnerabilities lead to contamination of food items.
3. Delineate the factors associated with an intentional contamination event.
4. Describe the three main purposes of foodborne disease surveillance.
5. Explain why many foodborne disease outbreaks go undetected.

Key Terms

epidemiologic investigation: Establishes the existence of an outbreak, confirms the diagnosis, and establishes the case definition and count cases.

foodborne disease outbreak (FBDO): Defined by the Centers for Disease Control and Prevention (CDC) as an incident in which two or more persons experience a similar illness, and food is implicated.

outbreaks of known etiology: Outbreaks for which laboratory evidence of a specific agent is obtained, and specified criteria are met.

outbreaks of unknown etiology: Outbreaks for which epidemiologic evidence implicates a food source, but adequate laboratory confirmation is not obtained.

traceback investigations: Identifies the source(s) of contamination to limit a public health threat by removing the source(s).

Introduction

The attacks of September 11, 2001 by al-Qaeda terrorists and the subsequent anthrax attacks have forced Americans to acknowledge their vulnerability to terrorism. As a result, improvements have been made by the US government and state agencies to combat terrorism and criminal acts against US infrastructures. However, according to many experts, the agricultural and food infrastructures remain highly vulnerable to both intentional and unintentional disruption (Chalk, 2004; Cupp, 2004; Monke, 2004). Tommy Thompson, former secretary of the US Department of Health and Human Services (HHS), expressed concern about the possibility of a terrorist attack against the nation's food supply during his resignation speech in 2004, and an attack on the agricultural and food infrastructures is more than a passing interest to terrorist groups (Peters, 2004). Hundreds of US agricultural documents that had been translated into Arabic were seized in Afghanistan following the US invasion of that country. Many experts agree that the threat of bioterrorism against the US agricultural and food infrastructures is growing and that the nation is not adequately prepared to handle such an attack (Chalk, 2003; Dyckman, 2003; Pear, 2004). According to these experts, there are several key vulnerabilities within the agricultural and food infrastructures, which make them a likely target of a bioterrorist attack.

Key Vulnerabilities in the Food Supply

The US agriculture and food infrastructures have features that make them vulnerable to both intentional and unintentional contamination. For example, the infrastructures are often concentrated. Domestic livestock and poultry are bred and reared in close proximity to one another in highly crowded populations (Chalk, 2003; Pear, 2004). An average-sized US dairy farm, for example, has between 1500 to 10,000 lactating cows at any one time. An average-sized hatchery has flocks as large as 350,000 hens or more (Perry, Banker, & Green, 1999). The sheer size and scale of these operations precludes farmers from attending to their animals on an individual basis (Chalk, 2004; Pear, 2004). Instead, they usually resort to the use of aggregate statistics, such as total milk yields, to monitor and regulate the health and well-being of their livestock or poultry. Also, these conditions increase the odds that a contagious disease, especially one that is airborne, would go undetected and spread rapidly (Chalk, 2004).

The homogeneous nature of the livestock and poultry industry also makes it vulnerable to an attack. Because the United States has not experienced a major foreign animal disease outbreak in livestock or poultry in more than 20 years, our animals have little or no innate resistance to these pathogens (Chalk, 2004; Cupp, 2004). Changes in husbandry practices and biotechnology innovations used to increase the quality and quantity of livestock/poultry and crop production have also led to an increase in susceptibility to pathogenic agents (Chalk, 2004; Pear, 2004). Modifications, such as sterilization programs, dehorning, branding, hormone injections, and use of antibiotics, increase stress levels and lower the natural tolerance of animals to disease from contagious organisms. Also, for both animals and crops, there are many foreign agents readily available in nature, from low-security laboratories, even from commercial sources, that require little effort and pose no risk to the health of the perpetrator. Terrorists might feel some sense of security in handling and dispersing these pathogens. When released, the bioterrorist event might go unnoticed for days to weeks, and it might be nearly impossible to determine if the event was manmade or occurred naturally. To further exacerbate the situation, the possible scenarios for deliberate contamination, even for unintentional contamination, are essentially limitless, and information on many of the potential targets and vectors is lacking.

The general lack of physical security and robust surveillance systems on many farms as well as in processing and packing plants also play an important role (Chalk, 2004; Monke, 2004). According to Chalk, the majority of the agricultural community has simply not thought about, much less physically sought to guard itself against, a deliberate act of sabotage. Outlying fields and feedlots seldom have extensive means to prevent access to unauthorized personnel, and the high turnover rate among workers in the agricultural and food industries creates a challenge for monitoring personnel security. Many of these workers are immigrants, and systems designed to ensure the authentication of these workers are still not in place. The scale and openness of the agricultural and food infrastructures, combined with the overall lack of security, provides numerous entry points for contamination to occur.

The problem is made worse by the rapid movement of vast amounts of product over broad geographies and through many hands from farm to fork (Chalk, 2004; Cupp, 2004). According to one survey of US barn auctions, 20% to 30% of cattle are regularly dispatched to locations at least 30 miles from their original point of purchase and, in many cases, they cross several states within 36 to 48 hours of leaving the sales yard. The rapid transfer of livestock increases the likelihood that pathogenic agents will spread well beyond the original site of a specific outbreak before health officials become aware that a problem exists (Chalk, 2004; Cupp, 2004). Many farms fail to quarantine new animals prior to introduction into the herd or flock. To further exacerbate the situation, the United States receives a wide range of imports from around the world. Approximately 1% of the foods imported into the United States are inspected at the borders prior to gaining entry.

Finally, the current US disease-reporting system does little to promote early warning and identification of pathogenic outbreaks (Chalk, 2004; Dyckman, 2003). Responsibility for reporting occurrences of livestock and poultry diseases lies with the agricultural producers; however, producers are reluctant to report outbreak occurrences for several reasons. First, channels of communication with the appropriate regulatory agencies or primary or secondary personnel are often confusing and rudimentary. Second, there are no standardized and consistent programs to compensate producers affected by a pathogenic outbreak because indemnity payments are usually determined on a case-by-case basis. For example, the 1999 Emergency Supplemental Appropriations Act provides less than 1% of the budgeted amount for livestock indemnity payments. Programs that provide compensation to farmers for depopulation of herds are usually for more common diseases, such as tuberculosis. For example, the Animal and Plant Health Inspection Service (APHIS) has implemented changes to the tuberculosis eradication program in the United States to include payment of indemnity for the depopulation of herds affected by tuberculosis. Furthermore, farmers might not

> **Learning Point:** Vulnerabilities of the US food supply:
>
> - Domestic livestock and poultry are bred and reared in close proximity to one another in highly crowded populations.
> - Animals have little or no innate resistance to pathogens that might be used in an attack.
> - There is a general lack of physical security and robust surveillance systems on many farms as well as in processing and packing plants.
> - There is rapid movement of vast amounts of product over broad geographies and through many hands from farm-to-fork.
> - The current US disease-reporting system does little to promote early warning and identification of pathogenic outbreaks.

want to invite quarantine and disease management officials onto their premises because of the perceived message it could send to the surrounding community.

Clearly, the methods used by the US agricultural and food systems to increase productivity and efficiency also contribute to the increase in vulnerability to a biological attack (Chalk, 2004; Cupp, 2004; Pear, 2004). Taking advantage of these vulnerabilities in these infrastructures would not require a significant undertaking, and there is a large menu of environmentally hardy pathogenic agents and chemical agents from which to choose. Also, there are many points at which either intentional or unintentional contamination could occur:

- on the farm (e.g., field crops or farm animals)
- during processing
- during distribution
- during storage
- at wholesale and retail food outlets
- in the home

Depending on the point at which the contamination occurred, the effects could be devastating, causing sickness or even death in a large number of persons, creating an atmosphere of anxiety and panic, causing disruption of the food distribution system, and/or damaging the agricultural economy (which makes up approximately

17% of the gross domestic product). Even a hoax has the ability to create anxiety and panic, disrupt food distribution, and damage the agricultural economy.

To further exacerbate the situation, the public health system is complex, and responsibilities for prevention and control can overlap or fall in the gray area between authorities of different agencies. Public health resources to assist industry and to coordinate effective preparedness and response strategies at the local, state, and federal levels are limited. Concerns about government overregulation and the proprietary nature of information within various food industries create barriers to effective sharing of information and coordination of emergency responses. Recognition of a foodborne bioterrorism attack can be delayed because of background levels of foodborne disease and potential widespread distribution of a contaminated product or ingredient. Systems for coordinated emergency response/crisis management between industry and government might not be adequate to deal with a serious threat to the food system. Rapid diagnostic methods for identifying bioterrorism agents in food are not consistently available, and coordinated laboratory systems for detection are not fully operational. Rapid traceback procedures for potentially contaminated products are not consistently in place.

> **Learning Point:** Because the United States has not experienced a major foreign animal disease outbreak in livestock or poultry in more than 20 years, our animals have little or no innate resistance to these pathogens.

Recognition of Foodborne Illnesses Associated with Intentional Contamination

The intentional release of a biological agent might not have an immediate impact due to the delay between exposure and illness onset (Kosal & Anderson, 2004). Also, outbreaks associated with intentional releases might closely resemble naturally occurring outbreaks. Such was the case in the 1984 outbreak of *Salmonella* serotype Typhimurium (ST) among 751 persons who ate at various restaurants in The Dalles, a small town in Oregon. Initially, public health officials classified this outbreak as an unintentional contamination. It was not until a year later that the leader of a cult known as Rajneeshee announced that the outbreak had deliberately been caused by some of his followers.

Several factors are indicative of an intentional release of a biological agent, including the following:

- an unusual temporal or geographic clustering of illness, such as illness occurring in persons attending the same public event or gathering (e.g., the 1984 *S. typhimurium* outbreak in The Dalles, Oregon)
- patients presenting with clinical signs and symptoms that suggest an infectious disease outbreak, such as two or more patients presenting with an unexplained febrile illness associated with sepsis, pneumonia, respiratory failure, or rash, especially if the illness occurs in otherwise healthy persons (e.g., the 2001 anthrax attack)
- an unusual age distribution for common diseases, such as an increase in what appears to be a chickenpox-like illness in adults
- a large number of cases of acute flaccid paralysis with prominent bulbar palsies, suggestive of a release of botulinum toxin

Although it was not a foodborne disease outbreak (FBDO), the 2001 anthrax attack demonstrated a pattern of illnesses and diagnostic clues indicative of an intentional release of a biological agent.

Cases of Intentional Contamination Involving Food Items in the United States

According to the Weapons of Mass Destruction (WMD) Database compiled by the Center for Nonproliferation Studies at the Monterey Institute of International Studies, there have been 31 cases of terrorism involving agriculture, crops, or food commodities as of March 2004 (Kosal & Anderson, 2004). Twenty of these cases were directed at crops and food commodities, and 10 were directed at livestock.

Additional cases were compiled in a database by Mohtadi and Murshid (2006). They identified approximately 85 cases of food contamination from several sources, including the WMD Database. The Mohtadi and Murshid database contained information on all terrorist-related activities and criminal acts, as well as events that were planned but not carried out, accounting for the increased number of events. All terrorist-related activities and criminal acts, as well as events that were planned but not carried out, have been included in this summary. However, discussion of these events has been limited to only those events occurring in the United States. For the purposes of this chapter, the events have been separated into three groups: events perpetrated by two or more individuals, events perpetrated by one individual, and events perpetrated by unknown individual(s). Fortunately, the US agriculture and food sectors have been fairly secure from deliberate contamination. Many of the recorded incidents were perpetrated by a single individual with criminal intent against a single person or a small group of people. Very few attacks have been perpetrated by a group with terrorist intent, and only one resulted in relatively large scale illness (1984 cult).

> **Learning Point:** There have been 31 cases of terrorism involving agriculture, crops, or food commodities as of March 2004.

Intentional Acts of Contamination Perpetrated by Two or More Individuals

Several groups committed acts of terrorism for political reasons. For example, in November 1970, a group known as the Weathermen allegedly attempted to acquire biological agents from a research facility in Frederick, Maryland (Mohtadi & Murshid, 2006). They allegedly planned to use these biological agents to contaminate the water systems of US urban centers to create public fear and bring about antigovernment sentiment. In January 1972, members of the right-wing group Order of the Rising Sun (RISE) were arrested in Chicago (Mohtadi & Murshid, 2006). The group possessed approximately 35 kg of typhoid cultures at the time of their arrest. According to sources, the agent was to be used to poison the water supplies in Chicago, St. Louis, and other Midwest cities. In 1984, a cult known as Rajneeshee contaminated the salad bars at several Oregon restaurants with *Salmonella* bacteria, resulting in at least 751 illnesses (Kosal & Anderson, 2004). The goal of the cult was to sicken enough registered voters to keep them from voting in an upcoming election. Cult members were upset with the county government for previously ruling against the cult in several real estate zoning disputes. Initially, public health workers classified this outbreak as an unintentional contamination. However, one year after the outbreak, the leader of the cult announced that the outbreak had been deliberately caused by some of his followers. As a result of an investigation into the matter, several cult members were eventually arrested and sentenced to jail terms.

Other groups commit acts of terrorism for racist reasons. For example, in March 1970, members of the Ku Klux Klan allegedly poisoned the water supply that served a 1000-acre farm that was owned and operated by a group of Muslims with cyanide, which resulted in the death of 30 cows and caused sickness in nine others (Cameron & Pate, 2001). In 1986, FBI agents raided a compound of a group called the Covenant, Sword and Arm of the Lord (CSA) (Mohtadi & Murshid, 2006). The cult, which was founded in 1971 by a former fundamentalist minister, James Ellison, was a paramilitary survivalist group with anti-Semitic and racist ideals. The raid by the FBI yielded a large quantity of weapons, including bombs and antitank rockets as well as significant quantities of potassium cyanide. According to one of the cult members, the potassium cyanide was to be used to contaminate the water supply of major US cities.

In other cases, the reason for acts of terrorism is not completely clear. For example, in 1983, the FBI arrested two brothers for producing an ounce of pure ricin. According to an informant, the brothers intended to contaminate the food and water supply with the ricin (Mohtadi & Murshid, 2006). In September 2000, two Jacksonville, Florida seventh graders allegedly contaminated the school cafeteria's salsa with rat poison, resulting in 34 cases of illness (Pate, Ackerman, & McCloud, 2001). In May 2000, three Rochester, New York teenagers were arrested and accused of tampering with food served at a fast food restaurant where they were employed. Allegedly the three teenagers contaminated food with bodily fluids and cleaning agents, including oven cleaner, over the course of eight months, from September 1999 to April 2000 (Pate, Ackerman, & McCloud, 2001). In October 2000, a small group of East Montpelier, Vermont students allegedly placed rat poison pellets in rice that was to be cooked for a home economics class (Pate, Ackerman, & McCloud, 2001).

Intentional Acts of Contamination Perpetrated by One Individual

There have been several cases of intentional contamination by a solitary perpetrator. Most of these events were small in nature and aimed at specific individuals or companies. For example, in October 1961, an outbreak of hepatitis A infection in 23 persons was traced to contaminated potato salad at an officers' mess hall in Florida (Carus, 1998). Although never confirmed, it was believed to have been an intentional contamination.

In April 1985, a man attempted to contaminate the New York City water supply with plutonium trichloride (Mohtadi & Murshid, 2006). His goal was to have murder charges dropped against Bernard Goetz, the "Subway Vigilante" who had shot four young African American men who were intent on robbing him on an express subway in Manhattan in 1984. While trace levels were detected in the water, plutonium emits alpha particles and is largely insoluble. Therefore, a very large quantity of plutonium would be needed to cause illness or death.

In June 1989, a member of a cleaning crew who worked for the FDA in New York stole a small amount of cyanide from the laboratory and used it to contaminate a departmental water cooler (Mohtadi & Murshid, 2006). An electrician who worked at the facility drank water from this cooler and became sick; he was then treated for his injuries and made a full recovery.

In December 1996, an anonymous letter was sent to the police chief of Berlin, Wisconsin indicating that feed products at the National By-Products Inc. had been tainted with pesticide and that the police should expect "large-scale animal mortality" (Mohtadi & Murshid, 2006). National By-Products Inc. is a supplier for the Purina Mills animal feed plant in Fond du Lac, Wisconsin. Purina feed was tested and found to contain low levels of contamination (one or two parts per million) on January 2, 1997. The following day, Purina stopped a shipment of 300 tons of feed bound for eastern and southern Wisconsin, as well as Illinois, Iowa, and Michigan. Officials from the Wisconsin Department of Agriculture, Trade and Consumer Protection announced that tallow at National By-Products Inc. had been deliberately contaminated with chloradane, a pesticide used to kill termites and that has been linked to cancer in humans. On September 14, 1999, the perpetrator was indicted for product tampering, and police investigation revealed that he had twice contaminated the plant's materials (Neher, 1999). The perpetrator owned a rival milk ranch, dead livestock removal company, and an animal food processing facility. The tainted feed had been distributed to over 4000 farms, principally dairies, and led to recalls in four Midwestern states of products, including cheese, butter, and ice cream, that were suspected of contamination as a result. The cost to the feed producer alone was estimated at over $250 million. Five months later, in May 1997, the same individual allegedly contaminated feed used for poultry with a fungicide (Neher, 1999). In both cases, letters were sent to customers indicating that tampering had taken place.

In 1996, 12 employees of a Dallas, Texas hospital became ill after consuming pastry that had been left in the laboratory's lunchroom (Mohtadi & Murshid, 2006). The pastries had been left there by a laboratory technician who had access to the *Shigella* cultures. The laboratory technician was indicted in August 1997 on three charges of tampering with food and was sentenced to 20 years in prison (Carus, 1998).

In August 1999, a Prince Frederick, Maryland woman laced soda cans with Drano in an effort to poison coworkers at a mental institution because she felt the workers mistreated the patients at the facility (Cameron & Pate, 2001).

In September 2000, a Jackson, Michigan ice cream stand worker allegedly poisoned the whipped cream he served to customers (Pate, Ackerman, & McCloud, 2001).

In January 2003, the CDC reported that 92 persons became ill after purchasing ground beef from a Michigan supermarket that had been intentionally contaminated with nicotine (Kosal & Anderson, 2004). A disgruntled employee of the supermarket that sold the contaminated meat was indicted for intentionally poisoning the 200 pounds of ground beef with an insecticide known as "black leaf 40."

In April 2003, 16 persons at a Maine church suffered from acute poisoning and one man died as a result of drinking coffee and eating snacks that had been contaminated with arsenic. An investigation revealed that the incident was a botched suicide attempt (Mohtadi & Murshid, 2006).

Intentional Acts of Contamination by Unknown Perpetrator(s)

The perpetrators of several contamination events have never been identified, nor have the reasons for the attacks. For example, in 1981, an unknown individual added organophosphate pesticide to a farm silo that was filled with cattle feed (Neher, 1999).

In 1982, seven persons in the Chicago area died after ingesting Tylenol capsules that had been contaminated with cyanide (Howard, et al, 1991). In March 1989, the US Embassy in Santiago, Chile received a call from an unidentified person claiming that grapes exported to the United States and Japan had been tainted with cyanide (Mohtadi & Murshid, 2006). The US Food and Drug Administration (FDA) immediately responded and located two grapes that had been contaminated with cyanide, which, due to the small quantity, posed no threat to human health. Responding to the incident, the United States, Japan, Germany, Canada, and Denmark halted Chilean fruit imports. This hoax demonstrated the potential impact of an attack against the food supply. Chile claimed losses of US$300 million, while US importers reported a financial windfall in excess of US$100 million. In February 1991, three persons in Washington became ill, two of whom died, after ingesting Sudafed capsules that had been laced with cyanide (Howard et al, 1991). In December 1999, seven students at a Springfield, Massachusetts law school became ill after drinking water from a cooler that had been contaminated with potassium cyanide. Members of the faculty and staff at the school suspected a connection between this incident and swastika-like graffiti around the water cooler (Cameron & Pate, 2001).

In October 2000, seven employees of a Hernando, Tennessee company were hospitalized after drinking coffee that was contaminated with rat poison (Pate, Ackerman, & McCloud, 2001).

In October 2003, a perpetrator going by the name "fallen angel" left a vial of ricin at a postal facility with a note threatening to dump ricin into the national drinking water supply unless new legislation dictating working hours for truck drivers was enacted (Mohtadi & Murshid, 2006). The FBI investigated the incident, but the perpetrator was never identified. In 2004, Gerber's baby food was discovered to be contaminated with ricin (Kosal & Anderson, 2004). Several containers contained a note stating that they had been contaminated with ricin. An FBI investigation into the matter found trace amounts of ricin in two jars of Gerber's baby food. The perpetrator(s) had evidently placed ground up castor beans with trace amounts of ricin in jars of the baby food. No arrests have been made, and it is unlikely that it could have led to serious injury due to the small amount present in the jars.

These cases highlight the ease with which the perpetrators were able to obtain and use biological agents. These unconventional forms of attack cause more fear than devastation and have the potential for more long-term effects, such as consumer fear, lack of trust in the ability of the government to protect its citizens, and economic consequences.

Naturally Occurring Foodborne Disease in the United States

Foodborne diseases are much more of a concern to government and the food industry today than a few decades ago (Todd, 1997). The identification of new agents that cause life-threatening conditions and the finding that traditional agents that were of no previous concern are being associated with food have contributed to the growing concern. An increasing number of large outbreaks are being reported, many of which have a considerable impact on children, the aging population, and persons with compromised immunity. Some of the other factors that have led to the growing concern include the ease of worldwide shipment of fresh or frozen food; the growing demand for traditional foods by immigrant populations; the growing demand for a wider variety of foods; and the development of new food industries, such as aquaculture. Reporting of these diseases is crucial to the development of prevention and response initiatives.

Reporting of Foodborne Disease Outbreaks (FBDOs) in the United States

Reporting of foodborne disease outbreaks (FBDOs) in the United States began more than a half century ago due to concern about the high morbidity and mortality caused by typhoid fever and infantile diarrhea (Bean, Goulding, Lao, & Angulo, 1996; Olsen, et al., 2004).

The goal was to obtain information about the role of food, milk, and water in outbreaks of intestinal illness to establish public health initiatives. In 1923, the Public Health Service began publishing summaries of outbreaks of gastrointestinal illness attributed to milk; outbreaks caused by all foods were added to summaries in 1938. These summaries helped lead to the enactment of important public health measures that had a profound impact on the incidence of enteric diseases, especially those transmitted by milk and water. From 1951 to 1960, the National Office of Vital Statistics reviewed reports of outbreaks of foodborne illness and published summaries annually in Public Health Reports. In 1961, the CDC assumed responsibility for foodborne disease surveillance and publishing reports on FBDOs.

Foodborne disease surveillance serves three main purposes (Bean, et al., 1996; Olsen, et al., 2004). The first is disease prevention and control. The three main prevention and control measures include the following:

1. early identification and removal of contaminated products from the commercial market
2. correction of faulty food-preparation practices in food-service establishments and in the home
3. rapid identification and appropriate treatment of human carriers of foodborne pathogens

The second purpose of foodborne disease surveillance is the acquisition of knowledge of disease causation. The responsible pathogen was not identified in over half of the FBDOs reported to the CDC between 1983 and 1987, which is similar to that of earlier years. In many of these outbreaks, pathogens known to cause foodborne illness are not identified due to late or incomplete laboratory investigations. In others, the pathogen responsible evades detection even after a thorough laboratory investigation due to a lack of information relating to the pathogen's role in FBDOs or because the pathogen simply could not be identified by available laboratory techniques. Identification of the causative agent has improved with the discovery of better viral diagnostic techniques; however, many agents still go unidentified.

The third main purpose of foodborne disease surveillance is administrative guidance. According to the CDC, the collection of data from investigations of FBDOs permits the assessment of trends in the prevalence of etiologic agents and in vehicles of disease transmission and brings to light common errors in food handling. Therefore, these data allow local and state health departments and others involved in the implementation of food protection programs to be informed of factors involved in FBDOs. This knowledge brings a greater awareness of the most important food protection methods, better training programs, and more effective use of available resources. The quality of the data depends on a commitment to surveillance of this type by state and local health departments. A department's interest in foodborne disease and its investigation and laboratory capabilities are important determinants of the quality of the investigation. The likelihood that the findings of the investigation will be reported varies from one locality to another.

It is important, however, to remember that the number of outbreaks reported by surveillance systems is only a small fraction of the true number that occurs (Bean, et al., 1996; Olsen, et al., 2004). The likelihood that an outbreak will be reported depends on many factors, such as ease of recognition and ease of laboratory conformation, consumers' and physicians' awareness, an interest in diseases surveillance activities of state and local health agencies, and the motivation to report the incident. For example, large outbreaks, multistate outbreaks, restaurant-associated outbreaks, and outbreaks involving serious illness, hospitalizations, or deaths are much more likely to come to the attention of health authorities than cases of mild illness after a family event (Todd, 1997). Also, foodborne diseases that are characterized by short incubation periods, such as those caused by chemical agents or staphylococcal enterotoxin, are more likely to be recognized as common-source FBDOs than those diseases with longer incubation periods, such as hepatitis A. Outbreaks that involve less common pathogens, such as *Bacillus cereus* or *Giardia lamblia*, are less likely to be confirmed as a source of illness because these organisms are often not considered in the clinical setting or by epidemiologic and laboratory investigations of FBDOs (Todd, 1997). Finally, because many food vehicles contain a variety of ingredients, they are a source of confusion. These factors

Learning Point: The number of outbreaks reported by surveillance systems is only a small fraction of the true number that occurs.

combined make investigations of FBDOs both difficult and time con-suming, and the usual result is that a number of FBDOs go undiscov-ered and unreported.

Foodborne Disease Outbreaks (FBDOs) Caused by Unintentional Contamination

Prior to 1998, the average annual number of FBDOs reported to the CDC was 504 (range, 387 to 653) (Bean, et al., 1990; Bean, et al., 1996; Olsen, et al., 2004). In 1998, better surveillance techniques were available, and the average number of FBDOs reported to the CDC increased to 1329 (Gerberding, 2006). The average annual num-ber of cases per outbreak reported to the CDC prior to 1998 was 17,007 (range, 11,015 to 31,079). The average number of cases per outbreak during 1998 to 2002 was 25,674 (range, 24,894 to 27,258). Although improvements appear to have been made in surveillance during the 1998 to 2002 reporting period, in the majority of out-breaks (about 65%; range, 55.5% to 72.4%), the etiology was not determined. This finding highlights the need for continued improve-ment in epidemiologic and laboratory investigation techniques.

It is important to note the improvements in viral diagnostic abil-ity for the 1998 to 2002 reporting period (Gerberding, 2006). The proportion of outbreaks with known etiology attributable to viruses increased from an average of 5.3% (range, 2.2% to 10.1%) in the years prior to 1998 to an average of 31.8% (range, 16.1% to 41.7%) in the years between 1998 and 2002. Prior to 1998, it was under-stood that viruses (e.g., Norwalk and Norwalk-like viruses) were probably a much more important cause of FBDOs than was currently recognized; however, local and state public health laboratories often lacked the resources and expertise to diagnose viral pathogens. Ac-cording to the CDC, methods to diagnose viral agents are now in-creasingly available in some state laboratories and, therefore, outbreaks of viral etiology might be more likely to be identified and reported in the future.

Foodborne Disease Outbreaks (FBDOs) in the United States Between 1983 and 2006

There are many opportunities for food to become contaminated as it is produced and prepared (Todd, 1997). Many of these pathogens, such as *Salmonella* and *Escherichia coli*, are present in healthy animals (usually in the intestines) that are raised for food. As a result, meat and poultry carcasses can become contaminated during slaughter by contact with small amounts of intestinal contents. Similarly, fresh produce can be contaminated when washed or irrigated with water that is contaminated with animal manure or human sewage (Bean, et al., 1996). During food processing, other foodborne microbes and viruses, such as *Shigella* or hepatitis A, can be introduced from infected humans who handle the food, by cross-contamination from raw meat or poultry, or by contaminated equipment used to process the food. Even a food that is fully cooked can be contaminated if it comes in contact with other raw foods or drippings from raw foods that contain pathogens. Raw foods of animal origin are most likely to be contaminated (e.g., raw meat and poultry, raw eggs, unpasteurized milk, and raw shellfish). Foods that combine the products of many individual animals are particularly harmful, such as bulk raw milk, pooled raw eggs, or ground beef. Fresh produce consumed raw is also of particular concern due to the fact that washing decreases but does not eliminate contamination. These facts lead to a number of possible sources of food to serve as vehicles of transmission (Table 10.1).

Raw, unpasteurized milk has been the source of a number of outbreaks. Unpasteurized milk can harbor a variety of dangerous microorganisms including *Campylobacter* spp., *Salmonella* spp., *Staphylococci*, *Yersinia*, *Listeria monocytogenes*, *Mycobacterium bovis*, *Brucella*, and even rabies, and symptoms can range anywhere from stomach cramps to coma and death (Herndon, 2007; Thomas & Powell, 2002). While some people regularly consume raw, unpasteurized milk products with no ill effects, illnesses and deaths associated with the consumption of raw milk occur each year. The most at risk are children, the elderly, pregnant women, and anyone with a compromised immune system. Supporters of raw, unpasteurized milk, such as the Real Milk Campaign, claim that it has benefits for the consumer, the farmer, the cows, and the environment. Supporters believe that the lack of "friendly bacteria" in pasteurized milk can provide a better environment for health-harming microorganisms to flourish. However, the FDA and CDC point to the outbreaks for proof of the dangers associated with consumption of unpasteurized milk.

For example, in 1983 there were two outbreaks of gastrointestinal illness following consumption of unpasteurized milk (Blessing,

Table 10.1   Foodborne Illness Outbreaks

CDC 5-year reporting period	FBDOs		FBDOs of bacterial etiology		FBDOs of chemical etiology		FBDOs of parasitic etiology		FBDOs of viral etiology	
	# outbreaks	# cases	# outbreaks	# cases	# outbreaks	# cases	# outbreaks	# cases	# outbreaks	# cases
1983 to 1987	2397	91,678	600	50,304	232	1244	36	203	41	2789
1988 to 1992	2423	77,375	796	33,206	143	927	17	379	45	2359
1993 to 1997	2751	86,058	655	43,821	148	576	19	2325	56	4066
1998 to 2002	6647	128,370	1184	37,887	221	1140	23	630	709	28,274

Source: Information for this table was compiled from the 5-year FBDO summary reports published by the CDC in *Morbidity and Mortality Weekly Reports.*

et al., 1983). The first outbreak occurred following a visit by 60 first-grade students and three teachers to a Pennsylvania dairy farm. Thirty-one (49%) of the 63 visitors became ill after consuming cookies and small cups of unpasteurized milk. *Campylobacter jejuni* was found in the stool of the only child who was cultured. The second outbreak also occurred following a visit to a Pennsylvania dairy farm. Forty-three kindergarten children and two teachers were served cookies and unpasteurized milk while visiting the farm. Twenty-six (58%) of the 45 visitors became ill, and *Campylobacter jejuni* was found in both stools that were cultured. Illness was not associated with consumption of cookies, touching farm animals, or consuming raw milk from other sources or with the presence of animals in the home in either of the outbreaks.

In 1984, two outbreaks, one in Minnesota (more than 20 cases; CDC, 1984b) and one in California (12 cases; CDC, 1984a) were associated with consumption of unpasteurized milk. In 1992, an outbreak (16 cases) of *E. coli* O157:H7 infections associated with consumption of unpasteurized milk occurred in Oregon (Keene, et al., 1997). In 2001, an outbreak (75 cases) of *Campylobacter jejuni* infections associated with consumption of unpasteurized milk occurred in Wisconsin (Harrington, Archer, Davis, Croft, & Varma, 2002). The dairy implicated in this outbreak provided unpasteurized milk samples at community events and to persons who toured the farm. They also sold unpasteurized milk to customers through a cow-leasing program, in which persons paid an initial fee to lease part of a cow and in turn received the milk. The unpasteurized milk for their 36 cows was stored in a bulk tank.

In 2002, a multistate outbreak (62 cases) of *Salmonella* serotype Typhimurium infections associated with consumption of unpasteurized milk occurred in Illinois, Indiana, Ohio, and Tennessee (Holt, et al., 2003). Epidemiologic and traceback investigations implicated a dairy restaurant in Ohio as the source of the unpasteurized milk. As a result of this outbreak, the implicated dairy relinquished its license for selling raw milk. In 2005, an outbreak (18 cases) of *E. coli* O157:H7 infections associated with consumption of unpasteurized milk occurred in Washington and Oregon (Bhat, et al., 2007). The farm implicated also participated in a cow-leasing program, and the milk from the five cows was stored in a bulk tank. According to the CDC, 45 outbreaks of foodborne illness were associated with consumption of either unpasteurized milk or cheese made from unpasteurized milk (Herndon, 2007). So, despite public warnings on the hazards of consuming raw, unpasteurized milk, retail sales and dairy-associated infections continue.

Many FBDOs have also been associated with consumption of pasteurized milk. For example, 49 patients in Massachusetts acquired listeriosis from pasteurized milk in 1983 (Fleming, et al., 1985). Seven of the cases occurred in fetuses or infants and 42 cases occurred in immune-suppressed adults; 14 (29%) of the patients died. The milk associated with the outbreak came from a group of farms on which listeriosis in dairy cows was known to have occurred at the time of the outbreak. This outbreak raised serious questions about the ability of pasteurization to remove *L. monocytogenes* from contaminated raw milk. In 1985, an outbreak of ST infections occurred in the midwestern part of the United States (Olsen, et al., 2004). This was the largest single FBDO ever reported to the CDC and was associated with the consumption of low fat pasteurized milk produced by a Chicago dairy farm. The outbreak resulted in more than 150,000 illnesses, 2777 hospitalizations, and 14 deaths in six midwest states. Laboratory analysis confirmed the presence of ST in more than 16,000 of the 150,000 cases. An outbreak of *Yersinia enterocolitica* O:8 infections associated with pasteurized milk occurred in 1995 in Vermont and New Hampshire (Ackers, et al., 2000). Ten patients were identified during this outbreak, three of whom were hospitalized. Consumption of bottle pasteurized milk from a local dairy was associated with the illness. Because no deficiencies in the pasteurization procedures or equipment were detected, this outbreak likely resulted from postpasteurization contamination of the implicated milk. Investigation revealed dairy pigs as the most likely source of contamination through contact with water used to rinse milk bottles. According to Ackers et al., education of dairy owners regarding *Y. enterocolitica* and postpasteurization contamination is necessary to prevent future outbreaks.

Cheese has served as a vehicle of transmission for many FBDOs. Many of these outbreaks were associated with Mexican-style soft cheese that has been made from unpasteurized milk, and it demonstrated the need to educate immigrants, especially those of Hispanic descent, of the dangers of consuming products made with unpasteurized milk. For example, an outbreak of *Brucella melitensis* infections due to unpasteurized goat cheese occurred in Mexican immigrants in Texas in 1983 (Perkins, et al., 1983). Twenty-nine persons became ill, 14 were hospitalized, and one person died. The cheese was reportedly produced in Mexico and was purchased from unlicensed vendors who sold it from their cars. In another outbreak, which occurred in California, 142 cases of human listeriosis were reported from January 1 through August 15, 1985 (James, et al., 1985). Ninety-three (65.5%) of the cases occurred in pregnant Hispanic women or their offspring and 49 (34.5%) occurred in non-pregnant, mostly Hispanic adults. The fatality rate was 34%; 18 nonpregnant adults, 20 stillbirths/miscarriages, and 10 neonates died during this outbreak. The outbreak was associated with consumption of Mexican-style soft cheese (odds ratio, 5.5; 95% confidence interval, 1.2 to 26.2). Laboratory analysis confirmed the presence of *L. monocytogenes* in the brand of Mexican-style cheese associated with the outbreak. A recall of the product was issued in June, and the factory was closed. Investigation of the factory indicated that the cheese was commonly contaminated with unpasteurized milk. In 1998, an outbreak of *E. coli* O157:H7 linked to consumption of fresh cheese curds occurred in Wisconsin (Durch, et al., 2000). Fifty-five laboratory-confirmed cases were identified, 25 of which were hospitalized. Because curds are sold fresh, the curds must be made with pasteurized milk. However, the dairy that produced the curds inadvertently used unpasteurized cheddar cheese to make the fresh curds, which were then labeled "pasteurized" cheddar cheese curds and distributed and sold in six Wisconsin counties. This outbreak illustrates the hazards of using unpasteurized milk to produce commercial products and the effects of mislabeling. In another outbreak of listeriosis among Mexican immigrants in North Carolina in 2000, 13 cases were identified; 12 were women (11 were pregnant) and one was a 70-year-old man (Boggs, et al., 2001). Among the 11 pregnant women, there were five stillbirths, three premature deliveries, and three infected newborns.

MacDonald et al. (2005) recommended education as a means to prevent further outbreaks. They also recommended enforcing laws that regulate the sale of raw milk and dairy products by unlicensed manufacturers and making listeriosis a reportable disease in all states. Mexican-style soft cheese is a staple of the Latin American diet, especially among Mexican immigrants. This cheese is often made using unpasteurized milk in noncommercial, unregulated production and then sold door to door and in small markets that cater to Latin American consumers in the United States.

According to the CDC, eggs have consistently been linked as a vehicle of transmission for FBDOs, especially those associated with *Salmonella enteritidis* (SE). For example, undercooked eggs in a bread-pudding dessert caused an outbreak of SE infections among conventioneers who attended a banquet in an Illinois hotel in 1990 (Bean, et al., 1996). Eleven hundred persons became ill, and 147 of these persons were hospitalized. In 1993, an outbreak of SE linked to consumption of homemade ice cream occurred in Florida (Buckner, et al., 1994). Twelve cases of salmonellosis were identified during this outbreak: five children and seven adults. The ice cream recipe included six grade A raw eggs. Because no errors on the part of the food handler were detected, the US Department of Agriculture (USDA) attempted a traceback investigation; however, because the eggs had been purchased from two suppliers (one of which had bought mixed eggs from many different sources), the traceback investigation was terminated.

In 1994, another outbreak was linked to consumption of ice cream (Hennessy, et al., 1996). There were an estimated 224,000 cases of infection associated with this outbreak, making this one of the largest FBDOs in US history. An investigation concluded that the outbreak was the result of contamination of pasteurized ice cream premix during transport in tanker trailers that had previously carried unpasteurized liquid eggs that contained SE. In 1994, an outbreak of salmonellosis was linked to consumption of hollandaise sauce at a Washington, DC hotel (Levy, et al., 1996). Fifty-six persons developed diarrhea, 20 of whom were hospitalized. Although cultures of the sauce yielded SE, cultures of the pooled whole raw shell eggs used to make the sauce did not. A traceback of the implicated eggs identified two flocks in Pennsylvania as possible sources for the eggs. In 1995, approximately 70 residents and staff of an Indiana nursing home developed salmonellosis following consumption of baked eggs. An investigation revealed that inadequate cooking might have contributed to this outbreak because the eggs were not stirred while being baked, and the internal temperature was obtained from only one place in the pan. The implicated eggs were traced to a New York distributor who had received the eggs from at least 35 different flocks (Levy, et al., 1996).

During another outbreak in 1995, 28 cases of salmonellosis were linked to consumption of Caesar salad dressing at a New York wedding reception (Levy, et al., 1996). The Caesar salad dressing was prepared with 18 raw shell eggs, olive oil, lemon juice, anchovies, Romano cheese, and Worcestershire sauce at 11:30 a.m. and then held unrefrigerated at the catering establishment for two hours. It was then transported in an unrefrigerated van until delivered and served at the reception at 6:00 p.m. In 1997, 13 members of a Girl Scout troop in California developed salmonellosis after consuming food prepared in a private residence (Reporter, et al., 2000). Cheesecake, which was served during the dinner, was associated with the outbreak. The cheesecake contained raw egg whites and egg yolks that had been cooked in a double boiler until slightly thickened. An investigation of the farm that had supplied the eggs found SE contamination in environmental samples of manure, feed, and water. On the basis of these findings, the flock was depopulated to prevent further SE cases.

Also in 1997, 43 cases of SE illness were identified among 75 attendees at seven events (a workshop dinner, nursing home luncheon, and five meals in private residences) in Washington, DC (Reporter, et al., 2000). Lasagna was implicated as the source of the seven outbreaks because it was the only food item common to all events. The lasagnas were prepared commercially by a company in Maryland, using fully cooked meat or spinach sauce and a mixture of raw shell eggs, ricotta and mozzarella cheeses, and spices. Most, if not all, of the lasagnas had been made on the same day from a single batch of the egg-cheese mixture. A traceback investigation led to two egg processors; five of 13 poultry houses had environmental samples positive for SE. As a result of this outbreak, the manufacturer of the lasagna voluntarily switched to using pasteurized eggs in egg-containing foods.

Ensuring that eggs are sold soon after being produced and that they are kept refrigerated are important steps in reducing egg-associated SE illness in the home. On-farm control measures, however, are necessary to help reduce the incident of egg-related outbreaks.

Since about 1990, outbreaks associated with fresh produce have increased by nearly threefold and the number of cases per outbreak has increased nearly 10-fold (Vugia, et al., 2007). These outbreaks are usually attributed to fecal contamination during postharvest handling, shipping, or processing in circumstances that permit bacterial multiplication These outbreaks have also included a wide variety of produce, such as lettuce, alfalfa sprouts, cantaloupe, and tomatoes. Because vegetables and fruit are considered to be an important part of a heart-healthy diet and are demanded year-round by consumers, this is a major public health problem. Contributing to the dilemma is the fact that fresh produce is usually grown in one or two specific areas due to climate limitation and then widely distributed to the rest of the United States. Second, fresh produce is usually grown in natural habitats for many known bacterial reservoirs (e.g., birds, amphibians, reptiles). Third, most fresh produce is consumed in raw form, and eradication of pathogens is difficult without cooking.

Leafy greens, such as lettuce and spinach, have been associated with several outbreaks. In 1986, an outbreak (347 cases) of *Shigella sonnei* infections following consumption of lettuce occurred in Texas (Davis, et al., 1988). The outbreak occurred at several outlets of a fast-food restaurant chain. The implicated fast-food restaurants had received the lettuce from one plant. Epidemiologic investigation indicated that a food handler at the plant might have contaminated the lettuce. In June 1996, an outbreak (61 cases) of *E. coli* O157:H7 infection associated with consumption of lettuce occurred in Connecticut and Illinois (Hilborn, et al., 1999). The implicated lettuce was traced to a single grower–processor that was located adjacent to a small beef cattle operation. Free-range chicken also had access to both the cattle and lettuce fields. This was the first multistate outbreak of *E. coli* O157:H7 infections associated with consumption of lettuce, highlighting the emergence of lettuce as a vehicle for food-borne pathogens. In 2006, an outbreak (183 cases) of *E. coli* O157:H7 infections associated with the consumption of fresh spinach occurred in 26 states (CDC, 2006). The fresh spinach identified as the source of the outbreak was traced to three California counties (Monterey, San Benito, and Santa Clara). According to the CDC, concurrent collection of case exposure information by epidemiologists in the affected states and sharing of exposure information among states and CDC led to the rapid identification of the suspected food source and public health action.

Since 1995, there have been 15 outbreaks of *Salmonella* spp. and two outbreaks of *E. coli* O157:H7 infections associated with sprouts (Mohle-Boetami, et al., 2002). In 1995, an outbreak (more than 240 cases) of *Salmonella* infections occurred in the United States and Finland (Mahon, et al., 1997). A traceback investigation implicated more than nine growers, all of which had obtained alfalfa seeds from a single US supplier, which had allegedly mixed seeds from lots bought in Italy, Hungary, and Pakistan. It was concluded that the alfalfa sprouts were grown from seed contaminated with *Salmonella* serotype Stanley (SS). In 1997, an outbreak (108 cases) of *E. coli* O157:H7 infections following consumption of alfalfa sprouts occurred in Michigan and Virginia (Como-Sabetti, et al., 1997). All implicated alfalfa sprouts were traced to a single sprouting facility. Inspection of the facility failed to identify obvious unsanitary practices, and environmental swabs did not yield contamination. In 2001, an outbreak (23 cases) of *Salmonella* serotype Kottbus (SK) infections associated with consumption of alfalfa sprouts occurred in Arizona, California, Colorado, and New Mexico. SK is extremely rare in the United States, and this was the second outbreak of SK since 1985; the first outbreak was also associated with sprouts. Because alfalfa sprouts are a raw agricultural commodity, they can be contaminated with animal feces and harbor such pathogens as *Salmonella* or *E. coli* O157:H7 during growth, harvest, processing, storage, shipping, or sprouting. Studies have shown that organisms present on seeds can increase up to 10,000-fold during the sprouting process (Jaquette, Beuchat, & Mahon, 1996). Therefore, research is needed to identify effective methods of seed decontamination.

Cantaloupes and other melons have been implicated in numerous outbreaks since 1990 (Anderson, et al., 2002). For example, in 1990, a multistate outbreak (295 cases) of *Salmonella* serotype Chester (SC) infections was traced to cantaloupes imported from Mexico (Ries, Zaza, Langkop, Tauxe, & Blake, 1990). In 1991, an outbreak (more than 400 cases) of *Salmonella* serotype Poona (SP) associated with consumption of contaminated melons occurred in 23 states (Francis, et al., 1991). Illness was associated with consumption of presliced cantaloupe in fruit salads or from salad bars. A trace back of the cantaloupe identified two possible sources of the cantaloupe: Rio Grande Valley in Texas and Mexico. Three multistate outbreaks of SP infections associated with consumption of cantaloupes occurred in the spring of consecutive years during 2000 to 2002 (Anderson, et al., 2002). Once again, the cantaloupes had been imported from Mexico. After these outbreaks, the FDA conducted farm investigations in Mexico, issued press releases to warn consumers, placed implicated farms on detention, and conducted sampling surveys of imported cantaloupe. Five percent of the cantaloupe sampled was contaminated with *Salmonella*.

Salmonella has been linked to tomatoes since 1990, when *Salmonella* serotype Javiana (SJ) caused 176 illnesses in four midwestern states (Hedberg, et al., 1999). In 2004, three outbreaks (a total of 562 culture-confirmed cases) of *Salmonella* infections associated with consumption of Roma tomatoes occurred in the United States and Canada (Corby, et al., 2005). Two were multistate outbreaks and one occurred in Canada. For each of the outbreaks, the tomatoes were traced from restaurants back to distributors, packers, or growers in the United States. The traceback identified one field-packing operation and three packinghouses from three states as possible sources. Salmonellae can enter the tomato plant through its roots or flowers or through small cracks in the skin or stem scars (Guo, van Iersel, Chen, Brackett, & Beuchat, 2002). After it is inside a tomato, it is difficult to eradicate *Salmonella* without cooking. Because uncooked tomatoes are an integral and nutritious component of the daily diet in the United States, with about five billion pounds of market fresh tomatoes being consumed annually, contamination is a great concern. According to the CDC, tomato-associated *Salmonella* outbreaks have increased in frequency and magnitude in recent years, with a reported 1616 cases occurring in nine outbreaks between 1990 and 2004. Our current knowledge of mechanisms of tomato contamination and methods of eradication of *Salmonella* in the fruit are inadequate to fully define interventions that will ensure product safety.

Several other vegetables and fruits have served as vehicles of transmission. For example, in 1983, an outbreak (28 cases) of *Clostridium botulinum* infections associated with consumption of sautéed onions occurred in Illinois (Doughty, et al., 1984). This was one of the largest foodborne botulism outbreaks reported in the United States. Another large outbreak (58 cases) occurred in Michigan in 1977 and was associated with consumption of home-canned peppers at a restaurant. Botulism outbreaks are usually isolated incidents involving a small number of cases and are usually attributed to improperly preserved home-canned or home-processed foods.

In 1988, a large outbreak (3175 cases) of *Shigella sonnei* infections occurred among persons who ate a raw tofu salad at an outdoor music festival in Michigan in 1988 (Bean, et al., 1996). A large number of volunteers handled the ingredients, and ill food handlers apparently contaminated the salad during preparation. In 1989, an outbreak (99 cases) of staphylococcal food poisoning associated with consumption of canned mushrooms occurred in United States (Levine, et al., 1996). Samples taken from unopened cans of mushrooms, which were imported from China, tested positive for staphylococcal enterotoxin. Because staphylococcal enterotoxin is not inactivated by temperatures used in canning and cooking, the staphylococci most likely grew and produced enterotoxin in the mushrooms before canning, or staphylococci contaminated the mushrooms after canning, possibly through improperly formed seams.

In 1990, a multistate outbreak (51 cases) of hepatitis A caused by consumption of strawberries occurred in the United States. An investigation of the outbreak indicated that the strawberries were most likely contaminated by an infected employee before distribution. In 1998, an outbreak (more than 250 cases) of *Shigella sonnei* infection associated with consumption of fresh parsley occurred in multiple restaurants in the United States and Canada (Crowe, et al., 1999). According to the investigation, the parsley was chopped in the morning and left at room temperature before it was served to customers. The parsley was traced back to a farm in Mexico, and a field investigation found that the farm used municipal, unchlorinated water to chill the parsley immediately after harvest and for making ice with which the parsley was packaged for transport. In 2000, an outbreak of cyclosporiasis associated with consumption of imported raspberries occurred at a Pennsylvania wedding reception (Ho, et al., 2002). Fifty-four (68.4%) of the 79 guests and members of the wedding party became ill following the event. The wedding cake, which had a cream filling that included raspberries, was the food item most strongly associated with illness (multivariate relative risk, 5.9; 95% confidence interval, 3.6 to 10.5), and leftover cake tested positive for *Cyclospora*. The raspberries were traced back to Guatemala. This was the fifth year since 1995 that outbreaks of cyclosporiasis have been associated with Guatemalan raspberries.

In 2003, an outbreak (29 cases) of SE infections were associated with the consumption of raw almonds in the United States and Canada (Keady, et al., 2004). The implicated almonds were traced to a producer in California. California produces about 80% of the world's almonds and about 100% of the almonds sold in the United States. This is only the second outbreak of salmonellosis associated with tree nuts. The first outbreak was identified in 2001, when raw almonds were linked to SE infections in Canada.

In 2003, an outbreak (555 cases) of hepatitis A infections associated with consumption of green onions among patrons of a restaurant occurred in Pennsylvania (Wheeler, et al., 2005). No ill food service worker that was identified could have been the source of the outbreak due to the date of illness onset. According to the investigation, the green onions were likely contaminated in the distribution system or during growing, harvest, packing, or cooling. Although the source of contamination has not been identified, the green onions have been traced to one or more farms in Mexico.

In 2004, an outbreak (96 cases) of cyclosporiasis associated with consumption of snow peas occurred in Pennsylvania (Crist, et al., 2004). Findings from the epidemiologic and traceback investigations implicated raw Guatemalan snow peas as the probable source of the outbreak. This was the first documented outbreak of cyclosporiasis linked to consumption of snow peas.

Several other types of fresh produce, such as raspberries, basil, and lettuce, from various countries have been implicated as vehicles for cyclosporiasis outbreaks in the United States. As a natural, uncooked food product, vegetables and fruit have the potential to become contaminated with pathogenic agents at any point (i.e., preharvest, during harvest, postharvest, etc.) and transmit them to consumers. Thorough washing of all fruits and vegetables before consumption is highly recommended; however, because washing reduces but does not eliminate bacterial contamination, production and processing methods need to be designed to minimize the number of pathogenic microorganisms present in the finished product.

Fruit juices have been implicated as a vehicle of transmission in at least 15 outbreaks in the United States in this century involving pathogens such as *E. coli* O157:H7, *Cryptosporidium parvum*, and *Salmonella* spp. (Parish, 1997). In 1995, an outbreak (62 cases) of *Salmonella enterica* serotype Hartford infections occurred among persons visiting a theme park in Florida (Cook, et al., 1998). Orange juice was implicated as the food vehicle responsible for the outbreak. A traceback investigation implicated a small local citrus processing plant located in a community adjacent to the theme park. A site inspection of the facilities identified several deficiencies, such as cracks and holes in the walls and rodent and bird droppings. A buildup of precipitate was also observed on equipment used to process the juice.

In 1996, an outbreak of *E. coli* O157:H7 infections attributed to unpasteurized apple juice made by the largest commercial producer of fresh juice in the United States was identified as the source of an outbreak (Cody, et al., 1999a). Seventy cases were identified; 25 (36%) of which were hospitalized, 14 (20%) developed HUS, and one (1%) died. Apple juice produced on the same day accounted for almost all of the cases, and the source of contamination was suspected to be incoming apples. According to an investigation, three lots of apples could explain contamination of the juice; two originated from an orchard frequented by deer that were subsequently shown to carry *E. coli* O157:H7, and one contained decayed apples that had been waxed.

In 1999, a commercially distributed unpasteurized orange juice traced to a single processor that distributes widely in the United States was linked to an outbreak of *Salmonella* serotype Muenchen (SM) in 15 states and Canada (Boase, et al., 1999). All together, more than 200 cases were identified during this outbreak, and more than 20 were hospitalized; none died. Samples were collected from previously unopened containers of the unpasteurized orange juice, from a smoothie blender and juice dispenser at an outlet of restaurants in Washington and from the factory that produced the orange juice. All tested positive for SM. The factory tested positive for SM, as well as yielding *Salmonella* serotypes Javiana, Gaminara, Hidalgo, and Alamo. This is the second and largest *Salmonella* outbreak associated with unpasteurized orange juice. The acidic nature of orange juice (pH of 3.4 to 4.0) was believed to inhibit bacterial growth; however, investigations have demonstrated otherwise. According to research, *Salmonella* serotypes Gaminara, Hartford, Rubislaw, and Typhimurium can survive in orange juice for up to 27 days at pH 3.5 and 60 days at pH 4.1 (Parish, Narciso, & Friedrich, 1997).

In 2006, an outbreak (four cases) of *C. botulinum* infections associated with commercial carrot juice occurred in Georgia and Florida (Shuler, et al., 2006). The carrot juice was traced to a manufacturing plant in California. Samples taken from the homes of the patients tested positive for botulinum toxin; however, samples collected from the implicated manufacturing plant did not. Because botulinum toxin was found only in the bottle of carrot juice that was consumed by the patients, a lapse in refrigeration of the carrot juice bottle during transport or storage was suspected.

As a result of the magnitude and severity of outbreaks associated with unpasteurized fruit juices, the FDA proposed two new regulations (Cody, et al., 1999; Boase, et al., 1999). The first requires that all unpasteurized fruit and vegetable juices carry a warning label stating that the product has not been pasteurized and might contain harmful bacteria that can cause serious illness in children, the elderly, and persons with weakened immune systems. The second regulation would mandate the application of hazard analysis critical control point (HACCP) principles to fruit and vegetable juice processing. However, these guidelines do not apply to juice or products containing juice that are sold by the glass in retail establishments, and many consumers might be unaware that they are consuming unpasteurized fruit juice.

Consumption of raw or undercooked fish and shellfish is a recurrent source of foodborne illness, including sporadic cases (Balter, et al., 2006). The most commonly associated pathogens include *Vibrio parahaemolyticus*, *Vibrio vulnificus*, *Norovirus*, and hepatitis A. Although fish and shellfish harvest areas in the United States and Canada are continually monitored by state control agencies, many of the bacteria associated with fish and shellfish multiply rapidly and, thus, can increase the levels of contamination if not rapidly refrigerated after harvest. To further exacerbate the situation, a majority of fish and seafood consumed in the United States is imported from countries such as Indonesia, Vietnam, and Thailand, only a small portion of which is inspected. Many fishermen outside of the United States use what is known as the "long-line" fishing method. Using this method, caught fish might be held in water for up to 20 hours before being removed from the line. In 1983, an outbreak (20 cases) of Norwalk virus associated with consumption of raw clams occurred. In 1996, an outbreak (16 cases) of *Vibrio vulnificus* infections associated with consumption of raw oysters occurred in California (Mascola, et al., 1996). *V. vulnificus* is one of the most severe infections, with a case-fatality rate for *V. vulnificus* septicemia of about 50%. In 2006, an outbreak (177 cases) of *Vibrio parahaemolyticus* infections associated with consumption of raw shellfish occurred in New York, Oregon, and Washington (Balter, et al., 2006). Traceback investigations linked the contaminated oysters and clams to harvest areas in Washington and British Columbia.

FBDOs associated with errors in meat and poultry processing and/or errors in cooking are well documented. Significant advances in food safety have been implemented by several industries to reduce the incident of outbreaks, but complex food distribution channels and frequent employee turnover remain ongoing challenges.

Beef has been associated with many of these outbreaks. An outbreak of *Escherichia coli* O157:H7 infection associated with hamburger consumption in a Nebraska nursing home occurred in 1984. Thirty-four persons were ill, 14 were hospitalized, and four died. This was the third reported FBDO associated with this organism in the United States; the first two occurred in 1982. In 1985, a statewide outbreak of chloramphenicol-resistant *Salmonella newport* infection occurred in California. The outbreak was associated with consumption of ground beef. A traceback implicated a dairy farm that used chloramphenicol.

Between December 1992 and February 1993, 501 cases of *E. coli* O157:H7 were reported in Washington; 151 of which were hospitalized, and three died (Bell, et al., 1994). Epidemiologic investigation implicated hamburgers from a fast-food restaurant as the source of the outbreak. A meat traceback to investigate the source(s) of contamination revealed that cattle were probably colonized with *E. coli* O157:H7 and that their slaughter caused surface contamination of the meat (Tuttle, et al., 1999). According to Bell et al., this is the largest reported FBDO associated with errors in meat processing and cooking.

In 1994, an outbreak of ST infection linked to consumption of raw ground beef occurred in Wisconsin (Frazak, et al., 1995). There were 107 confirmed cases of ST and 51 probable cases, 17 of which were hospitalized. Consumption of raw ground beef was implicated as the cause of the outbreak (odds ratio, 28; 95% confidence interval, 7 to 117). Knowledge of previous reports of outbreaks related to consumption of raw or undercooked beef was less among ill persons than among controls in the case-control study (odds ratio, 0.6; 95% confidence interval, 0.2 to 1.8). According to epidemiologic investigation, inadequate cleaning and sanitization of the meat grinder was most likely responsible for the contamination of the ground beef during this outbreak.

In 1997, an outbreak (15 cases) of *E. coli* O157:H7 infections was associated with consumption of a nationally distributed commercial brand of frozen ground beef patties and burgers in Colorado (Shillam, Heltzel, Beebe, & Hoffman, 1997). A multistate outbreak of *E. coli* O157:H7 infection linked to consumption of beef tacos at a fast-food restaurant chain occurred in California, Nevada, and Arizona in 1999 (Jay, et al., 2004). The outbreak resulted in 13 illnesses, five hospitalizations, and three cases of HUS. A traceback investigation linked an upstream supplier of beef to the outbreaks; however, a farm investigation was not possible. This outbreak also highlighted the need for a more efficient tracking system for food products.

In 2002, an outbreak (18 cases) of *E. coli* O157:H7 infections occurred in the United States (Shillam, et al, 2002). An investigation of the outbreak identified ground beef purchased from a grocery chain as the source of the outbreak. *E. coli* O157:H7 was cultured from an opened package of ground beef collected from a patient's home. The traceback of the ground beef identified a nationwide beef distributor. On June 30, the company issued a nationwide recall of 354,000 pounds of ground beef products. In July, the USDA increased the recall to 18.6 million pounds of fresh and frozen ground beef and beef trimmings. Foods of bovine origin, particularly ground beef, are common sources of sporadic infections and outbreaks of *E. coli* O157:H7. Surveys conducted on feed lots demonstrate that cattle can be infected symptomatically with *E. coli* O157:H7, and the prevalence of *E. coli* O157:H7 in feed lots can reach 63% to 100% particularly during the summer, under muddy conditions, or with feeding of barley. The expanded recall announced on July 19 was one of the largest in US history.

Consumers should be aware that microbiological testing in meat processing plants cannot eliminate the risk for contamination of ground beef with *E. coli* O157:H7 and other pathogens and that the use of safe food preparation practices is the best method by which to protect themselves.

In 2004, a multistate outbreak (31 cases) of *Salmonella typhimurium* infections linked to consumption of ground beef occurred in the United States (Cronquist, et al., 2006). Epidemiologic and traceback investigations identified one common supplier as the source of the outbreak; however, plant processing practices appeared to adhere to current FSIS production guidelines.

Poultry has also been implicated in many outbreaks. For example, in 1982, two outbreaks (112 cases) of *Salmonella* infections due to improperly cooked poultry giblets occurred in Maine (Gensheimer, 1984). The giblets were used to make gravy, and leftover gravy in each outbreak tested positive for *Salmonella*. Culture surveys of both poultry flocks and market poultry have shown that salmonellae can be recovered frequently (Gensheimer, 1984). In 1986, an outbreak (67 cases) of *Staphylococcus aureus* infections associated with consumption of turkey occurred at a buffet in New Mexico (Munoz, et al., 1986). Culture samples of the turkey yielded *S. aureus*, and a review of food handling procedures indicated that the turkey had been cooled for three hours at room temperature, ample time for bacterial proliferation and toxin production to occur. An outbreak of *Salmonella* serotype Agona infections among conventioneers attending a buffet catered by a South Carolina restaurant was caused by improperly handled turkey meat in 1990. A total of 851 persons became ill; 18 of whom were hospitalized.

In 1998, an outbreak (40 cases) of listeriosis infections associated with consumption of hot dogs occurred in 10 states (CDC, 1998). Four deaths occurred, including one fetus and three elderly persons. In 2000, another multistate outbreak (29 cases) of listeriosis infections associated with consumption occurred (Hurd, et al., 2000). A case-control study conducted by five states and two local health departments and the CDC implicated consumption of deli turkey meat as the probable source of the infection. A traceback investigation of the deli turkey meat implicated a manufacturer in Texas. As a result of the outbreak, the company stopped shipping ready-to-eat foods and, on December 14, voluntarily recalled processed turkey and chicken deli meat that might have been contaminated.

An increasing number of outbreaks are associated with manufactured products. For example, in 1998, a large, multistate outbreak of *Salmonella* serotype Agona (SA) associated with toasted oat cereal occurred in the United States (CDC, 1998). A total of 209 illnesses occurred, and 47 people were hospitalized. A culture of an open box of the cereal obtained from the home of a patient yielded SA at the CDC, and the FDA isolated SA from two separate composite samples from unopened boxes. This outbreak represents the first time that a commercial cereal product was implicated in a *Salmonella* outbreak. Because *Salmonella* spp. are relatively resistant to desiccation, it can survive for long periods in dry environments such as that found in cereal.

In 1989, a multistate outbreak (162 cases) of staphylococcal food poisoning that was associated with canned mushrooms imported from China occurred in the United States (Bean et al., 1996). In 2003, an outbreak (18 cases) of ST infections associated with the consumption of commercially processed egg salad occurred in Oregon (Keene, Hedberg, Cieslak, Schafer, & Dechet, 2004). A traceback investigation implicated a California plant; however, the specific mechanism of contamination was undetermined. As a result of this outbreak, the California vendor voluntarily discontinued the product.

In 2006, an outbreak of *Salmonella* serotype Tennessee infections associated with consumption of manufactured peanut butter occurred in the United States. An epidemiologic study comparing foods that ill and well persons said they ate showed that consumption of Peter Pan peanut butter and Great Value peanut butter were both statistically associated with illness and therefore the likely source of the outbreak. Product testing confirmed the presence of the outbreak strain of ST in opened jars of peanut butter obtained from ill persons. Both brands of peanut butter were traced back to a single facility in Georgia. As of May 22, 2007, 628 cases of ST infection had been reported to the CDC from 47 states. This is the first foodborne disease outbreak in which peanut butter was the food vehicle in US history. This outbreak is important because it demonstrated the potential for widespread illness from a broadly distributed, contaminated product.

In 2007, an outbreak (4 cases) of botulism infections associated with commercially canned chili occurred in Texas and Indiana (Ginsberg, et al, 2007). Investigations conducted by state and local health departments revealed that all four patients had consumed the same brand of hot dog chili sauce. All four patients were hospitalized and required mechanical ventilation. Botulinum toxin type A was detected in the serum of one Indiana patient and in a leftover chili mixture obtained from his home. The manufacturing company subsequently recalled the implicated brand and several other products produced in the same set of retorts (commercial-scale pressure cookers for processing canned foods) at the same canning facility. An examination of the canning facility in Georgia during the outbreak investigation identified deficiencies in the canning process. As a result, the recall was expanded on July 21 to include all production dates for 91 types of canned chili sauce, chili, other meat products, chicken products, and dog food that were manufactured in the same set of retorts as the hot dog chili sauce. This was the first outbreak of foodborne botulism in the United States associated with a commercial canning facility in approximately 30 years.

Chapter Summary

Although improvements have been made by the US government and state agencies to improve prevention and response capabilities, the agricultural and food infrastructures remain highly vulnerable to both intentional and unintentional disruption. Several key vulnerabilities inherent in these infrastructures make them susceptible to contamination by both pathogenic and chemical agents. For example, the infrastructures are often highly concentrated and highly complex. Also, the homogenous nature of crops and livestock/poultry makes them vulnerable to foreign and reemerging diseases. There is also a general lack of physical security and robust surveillance systems on many farms as well as in processing and packing plants. The problem is made worse by the rapid movement of vast amounts of product over broad geographies and through many hands from farm-to-fork. Finally, the current US disease-reporting system does little to promote early warning and identification of pathogenic outbreaks, and the public health system is complex, with overlap or gray areas that can result in a lack of coordination.

Issues to Debate

1. What improvements could be made in the agriculture and food infrastructures to reduce the incidence of FBDOs?
2. How can you determine if an FBDO is due to an intentional attack or a naturally occurring event?
3. Which point during the food continuum is the most vulnerable and why?
4. Which food commodities are most prevalent in the literature, and why do you think this is the case?
5. What is the most common means of contamination of a food commodity, and why do you think this is the case?

References

Ackers, M., Schoenfeld, S., Markman, J., Smith, M. G., Nicholson, M. A., DeWitt, W., et al. (2000). An outbreak of *Yersinia enterocolitica* O:8 infections associated with pasteurized milk. *The Journal of Infectious Diseases, 181*, 1834–1837.

Anderson, S. M., Verchick, L., Sowadsky, R., Sun, B., Civen, R., Mohle-Boetani, J. C., et al. (2002). Multistate outbreaks of *Salmonella* serotype Poona infections associated with eating cantaloupe from Mexico—United States and Canada, 2000–2002. *Morbidity and Mortality Weekly Report, 51*, 1044–1047.

Balter, S., Hanson, H., Kornstein, L., Lee, L., Reddy, V., Sahl, S., et al. (2006). *Vibrio parahaemolyticus* infections associated with consumption of raw shellfish—Three states, 2006. *Morbidity and Mortality Weekly Report, 55*, 854–856.

Bean, N. H., Griffin, P. M., Goulding, J. S., & Ivey, C. B. (1990). Foodborne disease outbreaks, 5-year summary, 1983–1987. *Morbidity and Mortality Weekly Report, 39*, 15–57.

Bean, N. H., Goulding, J. S., Lao, C., & Angulo, F. J. (1996). Surveillance for foodborne-disease outbreaks—United States, 1988–1992. *Morbidity and Mortality Weekly Report, 45*, 1–55.

Bell, B. P., Goldoft, M., Griffin, P. M., Davis, M. A., Gordon, D. C., Tarr, P. I., et al. (1994). A multistate outbreak of *Escherichia coli* O157:H7-associated blood diarrhea and hemolytic uremic syndrome from hamburgers. The Washington experience. *The Journal of the American Medical Association, 272*, 1349–1353.

Bhat, M., Denny, J., MacDonald, K., Hofmann, J., Jain, S., & Lynch, M. (2007). *Escherichia coli* O157:H7 infection associated with drinking raw milk—Washington and Oregon, November–December, 2005. *Morbidity and Mortality Weekly Report, 56*, 165–167.

Blessing, D. J., Thompson, M., Fisher, B., Schooley, D., Kramer, M. J., DeMelfi, T. M., et al. (1983). Campylobacteriosis associated with raw milk consumption—Pennsylvania. *Morbidity and Mortality Weekly Report, 32*, 337–338, 344.

Boase, J., Lipsky, S., Simani, P., Smith, S., Skilton, C., Greenman, S., et al. (1999). Outbreak of *Salmonella* serotype Muenchen infections associated with unpasteurized orange juice—United States and Canada, June 1999. *Morbidity and Mortality Weekly Report, 48*, 582–585.

Boggs, J. D., Whitwam, R. E., Hale, L. M., Briscoe, R. P., Kahn, S. E., Forsyth, M. D., et al. (2001). Outbreak of listeriosis associated with homemade Mexican-style cheese—North Carolina, October 2000–January 2001. *Morbidity and Mortality Weekly Report, 50*, 560–562.

Buckner, P., Ferguson, D., Anzalone, F., Anzalone, D., Taylor, J., & Hopkins, R. S. (1994). Outbreak of *Salmonella enteritidis* associated with homemade ice cream—Florida, 1993. *Morbidity and Mortality Weekly Report, 43*, 669–671.

Cameron, G., & Pate, J. (2001). Covert biological weapons attacks against agricultural targets: Assessing the impact against US agriculture. *Terrorism and Political Violence, 13*, 61–82.

Carus, S. (1998). *Bioterrorism and biocrimes: The illicit use of biological agents since 1900*. Retrieved August 7, 2007, from http://www.fas.org

Chalk, P. (2003). *Agroterrorism: What is the threat and what can be done about it?* Retrieved August 10, 2007, from http://www.rand.org

Chalk, P. (2004). *Hitting America's soft underbelly: The potential threat of deliberate biological attack against the US agricultural and food industry*. Retrieved August 10, 2007, from http://www.rand.org

CDC. (1984a). Epidemiologic notes and reports *Campylobacter* outbreak associated with certified raw milk products—California. *Morbidity and Mortality Weekly Report, 33*, 562.

CDC. (1984b). Epidemiologic notes and reports chronic diarrhea associated with raw milk consumption. *Morbidity and Mortality Weekly Report, 33*, 521–522, 527–528.

CDC. (1998). Multistate outbreak of *Salmonella* serotype Agona infections linked to toasted oats cereal—United States, April–May, 1998. *Morbidity and Mortality Weekly Report, 47*, 462–464.

CDC. (2006). Ongoing multistate outbreak of *Escherichia coli* serotype O157:H7 infections associated with consumption of fresh spinach—United States, September 2006. *Morbidity and Mortality Weekly Report, 55*, 1045–1046.

Cody, S. H., Glynn, M. K., Farrar, J. A., Cairns, K. L., Griffin, P. M., Kobayashi, J., et al. (1999a). An outbreak of *Escherichia coli* O157:H7 infection from unpasteurized commercial apple juice. *Annals of Internal Medicine, 130*, 202–209.

Como-Sabetti, K., Reagan, S., Allaire, S., Parrott, K., Simonds, C. M., Hrabowy, S., et al. (1997). Outbreaks of *Escherichia coli* O157:H7 infection associated with eating alfalfa sprouts—Michigan and Virginia, June–July, 1997. *Morbidity and Mortality Weekly Report, 46*, 741–744.

Cook, K. A., Dobbs, T. E., Illady, G., Wells, J. G., Barrett, T. J., Puhr, N. D., et al. (1998). Outbreak of *Salmonella* serotype Hartford infections associated with unpasteurized orange juice. *The Journal of the American Medical Association, 280*, 1504–1509.

Corby, R., Lanni, V., Kistler, V., Dato, V., Weltman, A., Yozviak, C., et al. (2005). Outbreaks of *Salmonella* infections associated with eating roma tomatoes—United States and Canada, 2004. *Morbidity and Mortality Weekly Report, 54*, 325–328.

Crist, A., Morningstar, C., Chambers, R., Fitzgerald, T., Stoops, D., Deffley, M., et al. (2004). Outbreak of cyclosporiasis associated with snow peas—Pennsylvania, 2004. *Morbidity and Mortality Weekly Report, 53*, 876–878.

Cronquist, A., Wedel, S., Albanese, B., Sewell, C. M., Hoang-Johnson, D., Ihry, T., et al. (2006). Multistate outbreak of *Salmonella* Typhimurium infections associated with eating ground beef—United States, 2004. *Morbidity and Mortality Weekly Report, 55*, 180–182.

Crowe, L., Lau, W., McLeod, L., Ciebin, B., LeBer, C., Easy, R., et al. (1999). Outbreaks of *Shigella sonnei* infection associated with eating fresh parsley—United States and Canada, July–August 1998. *Morbidity and Mortality Weekly Report, 48*, 285–289.

Cupp, O.S., Walker, D. E., & Hillison J. (2004). Agroterrorism in the US: Key security challenges for the 21st century. *Biosecurity and Bioterrorism, 2*, 97–105.

Davis, H., Taylor, J. P., Perdue, J. N., Stelma, G. N., Rowntree, R., & Greene, K. D. (1988). A shigellosis outbreak traced to commercially distributed shredded lettuce. *American Journal of Epidemiology, 128*, 1312–1321.

Doughty, S. C., O'Connor, R. P., Alexander, J., Sidler, G. J., Churchill, S., Parker, J. W., et al. (1984). Foodborne botulism—Illinois. *Morbidity and Mortality Weekly Report, 33*, 22–23.

Durch, J., Ringhand, T., Manner, K., Barnett, M., Proctor, M., Davis, J., et al. (2000). Outbreak of *Escherichia coli* O157:H7 infection associated with eating fresh cheese curds—Wisconsin, June 1998. *Morbidity and Mortality Weekly Report, 49*, 911–913.

Dyckman, L. J. (2003). *Bioterrorism: A threat to agriculture and the food supply* [Testimony before the US Senate]. Retrieved August 7, 2007, from http://www.gao.gov

Fleming, D. W., Cochi, S. L., MacDonald, K. L., Brondum, J., Hayes, P. S., Plikaytis, B. D., et al. (1985). Pasteurized milk as a vehicle of infection in an outbreak of listeriosis. *New England Journal of Medicine, 14*, 404–407.

Francis, B. J., Altamirano, J. V., Stobierski, M. G., Hall, W., Robinson, B., Dietrich, S., et al. (1991). Epidemiologic notes and reports: Multistate outbreak of *Salmonella* Poona infections—United States and Canada, 1991. *Morbidity and Mortality Weekly Report, 40*, 549–552.

Frazak, P. A., Kazmierrczak, J. J., Procter, M. E., Davis, J. P., Larson, J., & Loerke, R. (1995). Outbreak of *Salmonella* serotype Typhimurium infection associated with eating raw ground beef—Washington, 1994. *Morbidity and Mortality Weekly Report, 44*, 905–909.

Gensheimer, K. F. (1984). Poultry giblet-associated salmonellosis—Maine. *Morbidity and Mortality Weekly Report, 33*, 630–631.

Gerberding, J. L. (2006). Pandemic preparedness: Pigs, poultry, and people versus plans, products, and practice. *Journal of Infectious Diseases, 194*, 77–81.

Ginsberg, M. M., Granzow, L., Teclaw, R. F., Gaul, L. K., Bagdure, S., Cole, A., et al. (2007). Botulism associated with commercially canned chili sauce, Texas and Indiana, July 2007. *Morbidity and Mortality Weekly Report, 56*, 1–3.

Guo, X., van Iersel, M. W., Chen, J., Brackett, R. E., & Beuchat, L. R. (2002). Evidence of association of *Salmonellae* with tomato plants grown hydroponically in inoculated nutrient solution. *Applied Environmental Microbiology, 68*, 3639–3643.

Harrington, P., Archer, J., Davis, J. P., Croft, D. R., & Varma, J. K. (2002). Outbreak of *Campylobacter jejuni* infections associated with drinking unpasteurized milk procured through a cow-leasing program—Wisconsin, 2001. *Morbidity and Mortality Weekly Report, 51*, 548–549.

Hedberg, C. W., Angulo, F. J., White, K. E., Langkop, C. W., Schell, W. L., Stobierrski, M. G., et al. (1999). Outbreaks of salmonellosis associated with eating uncooked tomatoes: Implications for public health. *Epidemiology and Infection, 122*, 385–393.

Hennessy, T. W., Hedberg, C. W., Slutsker, L., White, K. E., Besserr-Wiek, J. M., Moen, M. E., et al. (1996). A national outbreak of *Salmonella enteritidis* infections from ice cream. *The New England Journal of Medicine, 334*, 1281–1286.

Herndon, M. (2007). *FDA and CDC remind consumers of the dangers of drinking raw milk*. Retrieved August 12, 2007, from http://www.fda.gov/bbs/topics/NEWS/2007/NEW01576.html

Hilborn, E. D., Mermin, J. H., Mshar, P. A., Hadlerr, J. L., Voetsch, A., Wojtkunski, C., et al. (1999). A multistate outbreak of *Escherichia coli* O157:H7 infections associated with consumption of mesclun lettuce. *Archives of Internal Medicine, 159*, 1758–1764.

Ho, A. Y., Lopez, A. S., Eberhart, M. G., Levenson, R., Finkel, B. S., da Silva, A. J., et al. (2002). Outbreak of cyclosporiasis associated with imported raspberries, Philadelphia, Pennsylvania, 2000. *Emerging Infectious Diseases, 8,* 783–788.

Holt, J., Propes, D., Patterson, C., Bannerman, T., Nicholson, L., Bundesen, M., et al. (2003). Multistate outbreak of *Salmonella* serotype Typhimurium infections associated with drinking unpasteurized milk—Illinois, Indiana, Ohio, and Tennessee, 2002–2003. *Morbidity and Mortality Weekly Report, 52,* 613–615.

Howard, J., Pouw, T. H., Arnold, J., Logan, B., Koayashi, J. M., Davis, J., et al. (1991). Epidemiologic notes and reports cyanide poisoning associated with over-the-counter medication—Washington State, 1991. *Morbidity and Mortality Weekly Report, 40,* 167–168.

Hurd, S., Phan, Q., Hadler, J., Mackenzie, B., Lance-Parker, S., Blake, P. et al. (2000). Multistate outbreak of Listeriosis, United States, 2000. *Morbidity and Mortality Weekly Report, 49,* 1129–1130.

James, S. M., Fannin, S. L., Agee, B. A., Hall, B., Parker, E., Vogt, J., et al. (1985). Epidemiologic notes and reports listeriosis outbreak associated with Mexican-style cheese—California. *Morbidity and Mortality Weekly Report, 34,* 357–359.

Jaquette, C. B., Beuchat, L. R., & Mahon, B. E. (1996). Efficacy of chlorine and heat treatment in killing *Salmonella* Stanley inoculated onto alfalfa seeds and growth and survival of the pathogen during sprouting and storage. *Applied and Environmental Microbiology, 62,* 2212–2215.

Jay, M.T., Garrett, V., Mohle-Boetani, J.C., Barros, M., Farrar, J.A., Rios, R., et al. (2004). A multistate outbreak of *Escherichia coli* O157:H7 infection linked to consumption of beef tacos at a fast-food restaurant chain. *Clinical Infectious Diseases, 39,* 8–10.

Keady, S., Briggs, G., Farrar, J., Mohle-Boetani, J. C., O'Connell, J., Werner, S. B., et al. (2004). Outbreak of *Salmonella* serotype Enteritidis infections associated with raw almonds—United States and Canada, 2003–2004. *Morbidity and Mortality Weekly Report, 53,* 484–487.

Keene, W. E., Hedberg, K., Cieslak, P., Schafer, S., & Dechet, A. (2004). *Salmonella* serotype Typhimurium outbreak associated with commercially processed egg salad—Oregon, 2003. *Morbidity and Mortality Weekly Report, 53,* 1132–1134.

Keene, W. E., Hedberg, K., Herriot, D. E., Hancock, D. D., McKay, R. W., Barrett, T. J., et al. (1997). A prolonged outbreak of *Escherichia coli* O157:H7 infections caused by commercially distributed raw milk. *Journal of Infectious Diseases, 176,* 815–818.

Kosal, M. E., & Anderson, D. E. (2004). An unaddressed issue of agricultural terrorism: A case study on feed security. *Journal of Animal Science, 82,* 3394–3400.

Levine, W. C., Bennett, R. W., Choi, Y., Henning, K. J., Rager, J. R., Hendricks, K. A., et al. (1996). Staphylococcal food poisoning caused by imported canned mushrooms. *Journal of Infectious Diseases, 173,* 1263–1267.

Levy, M., Fletcher, M., Moody, M., Bur, M. S., Cory, D., Corbitt, W., et al. (1996). Outbreaks of *Salmonella* serotype Enteritidis infection associated with consumption of raw shell eggs, United States, 1994–1995. *Morbidity and Mortality Weekly Report, 45,* 737–742.

MacDonald, P. D., Whitwam, R. E., Boggs, J. D., MacCormack, J. N., Anderson, K. L., Reardon, J. W., et al. (2005). Outbreak of listeriosis among Mexican immigrants as a result of consumption of illicitly produced Mexican-style cheese. *Clinical Infectious Diseases, 40,* 677–682.

Mahon, B. E., Pönkä, A., Hall, W. N., Komatsu, K., Dietrich, S. E., Siitonen, A., et al. (1997). An international outbreak of *Salmonella* infections caused by alfalfa sprouts grown from contaminated seeds. *Journal of Infectious Diseases, 175,* 876–882.

Mascola, L., Tormey, M., Dassey, D., Kilman, L., Harvey, S., Medina, A., et al. (1996). Vibrio vulnificus infections associated with eating raw oysters, Los Angeles, 1996. *Morbidity and Mortality Weekly Report, 45,* 621–624.

Mohle-Boetami, J., Werner, B., Polumbo, M., Farrar, J., Vugia, D., Anderson, S., et al. (2002). Outbreaks of *Salmonella* serotype Kottbus infections associated with eating alfalfa sprouts—Arizona, California, Colorado, and New Mexico, February–April 2001. *Morbidity and Mortality Weekly Report, 51,* 7–9.

Mohtadi, H., & Murshid, A. (2006). *A global chronology of incidents of chemical, biological, radioactive, and nuclear attacks: 1950–2005.* Retrieved August 10, 2007, from http://www.ncfpd.umn.edu

Monke, J. (2004). Agroterrorism: Threats and preparedness [CRS report for Congress]. Retrieved August 7, 2007, from http://www.fas.org

Munoz, R., Ornelas, E., Nickey, L. N., Balcorta, S., Sublasky, D., Rivas, I., et al. (1986). Staphylococcal food poisoning from turkey at a country club buffet—New Mexico. *Morbidity and Mortality Weekly Report, 35,* 715–716, 721–722.

Neher, N. J. (1999). The need for a coordinated response to food terrorism: The Wisconsin experience. *Annuals of the New York Academy of Science, 894,* 181–184.

Olsen, S. J., Ying, M., Davis, M. F., Deasy, M., Holland, B., Iampietro, L., et al. (2004). Multidrug-resistant *Salmonella* Typhimurium infection from milk contaminated after pasteurization. *Emerging Infectious Diseases, 10,* 932–935.

Parish, M. E. (1997). Public health and nonpasteurized fruit juices. *Critical Reviews in Microbiology, 23,* 109–119.

Parish, M. E., Narciso, J. A., & Friedrich, L. M. (1997). Survival of *Salmonella* in orange juice. *Journal of Food Safety, 17,* 273–281.

Pate, J., Ackerman, G., & McCloud, K. (2001). *2000 WMD terrorism chronology: Incidents involving sub-national actors and chemical, biological, radiological, or nuclear materials.* Retrieved August 10, 2007, from http://cns.miis.edu/pubs/reports/cbrn2k.htm

Pear, R. (2004). *US Health Chief, stepping down, issues warning.* Retrieved August 6, 2007, from http://www.nytimes.com

Perkins, P., Rogers, A., Key, M., Pappas, V., Wende, R., Epstein, J., et al. (1983). Epidemiologic notes and reports brucellosis—Texas. *Morbidity and Mortality Weekly Report, 32,* 548–553.

Perry, J., Banker, D., & Green, R. (1999). *Broiler farms' organization, management, and performance.* Retrieved August 15, 2007, from http://www.ers.usda.gov

Peters, K. M. (2003). *Officials fear terrorist attack on US food supply.* Retrieved August 6, 2007, from http://www.govexec.com

Reporter, R., Mascola, L., Mohle-Boetani, J., Farrar, J., Vugia, D., Fletcher, M., et al. (2000). Outbreaks of *Salmonella* serotype Enteritidis infection associated with eating raw or undercooked shell eggs—United States, 1996–1998. *Morbidity and Mortality Weekly Reports, 49,* 73–79.

Ries, A. A., Zaza, S., Langkop, C., Tauxe, R. V., & Blake P. A. (1990). A multistate outbreak of *Salmonella* Chester linked to imported cantaloupe [Abstract No. 915]. In Program and Abstracts of the 30th Interscience Conference on Antimicrobial Agents and Chemotherapy. Washington, DC: American Society of Microbiology.

Shillam, P., Heltzel, D., Beebe, J., & Hoffman, R. (1997). *Escherichia coli* 0157:H7 infections associated with eating a nationally distributed commercial brand of frozen ground beef patties and burgers—Colorado, 1997. *Morbidity and Mortality Weekly Report, 46,* 777–778.

Shillam, P., Woo-Ming, A., Mascola, L., Bagby, R., Lohff, C., Bidol, S., et al. (2002). Multistate outbreak of *Escherichia coli* 0157:H7 infections associated with eating ground beef, United States, June–July 2002. *Morbidity and Mortality Weekly Report, 51,* 637–639.

Shuler, C., Drenzek, D., Lance, S., Gonzalez, G., Miller, J., Tobin-D'Angelo, M., et al. (2006). Botulism associated with commercial carrot juice—Georgia and Florida, September 2006. *Morbidity and Mortality Weekly Report, 55,* 1098–1099.

Thomas, K., & Powell, D. (2002). *Risks of raw milk.* Retrieved August 5, 2007, from http://www.foodsafety.ksu.edu

Todd, E. C. (1997). Epidemiology of foodborne deseases: A worldwide review. *World Health Statistics Quarterly, 50,* 30–50.

Tuttle, J., Gomez, T., Doyle, M. P., Wells, J.G., Zhao, T., Tauxe, R. V., et al. (1999). Lessons from a large outbreak of *Escherichia coli* 0157:H7 infections: Insights into the infectious dose and method of widespread contamination of hamburger patties. *Epidemiology and Infection, 122,* 185–192.

Vugia, D., Cronquist, A., Hadler, J., Tobin-D'Angelo, M., Blythe, D., Smith, K., et al. (2007). Preliminary FoodNet data on the incidence of infection with pathogens transmitted commonly through food. *Morbidity and Mortality Weekly Report, 56,* 336–339.

Wheeler, C., Vogt, T. M., Armstrong, G. L., Vaughan, G., Weltman, A., Nainan, O. V., et al. (2005). An outbreak of hepatitis A associated with green onions. *New England Journal of Medicine, 353,* 890–897.

CHAPTER 11

KEY ISSUES ASSOCIATED WITH FOODBORNE DISEASE OUTBREAKS

Tamara M. Crutchley Bushell, PhD

Chapter Objectives

After reading the chapter and reflecting on the contents, you should be able to:

1. Identify key factors inherent in the agricultural infrastructure that increase the likelihood of food contamination.
2. Describe the significance of pathogen carriage in livestock, poultry, and crops.
3. Understand why antibiotic-resistant bacteria is an important food safety issue.
4. Explain how globalization of the food supply increases the incidence of foodborne disease outbreaks.
5. Discuss how weaknesses in federal oversight of food safety affect the size and severity of foodborne disease outbreaks.

Key Terms

antibiotic resistance: A condition where microorganisms continue to multiply although exposed to antibiotic agents, often because the bacteria has become immune.

emerging pathogen: An organism, especially a microorganism, that has recently been recognized as a pathogen.

food security: Defined by the FAO (1996) as the state achieved when food systems operate such that "all people, at all times, have physical and economic access to sufficient, safe, and nutritious food to meet their dietary needs and food preferences for an active and healthy life."

food system: A set of dynamic interactions between and within the biogeophysical and human environments that result in the production, processing, distribution, preparation, and consumption of food (Gregory, Ingram, & Brklacich, 2005).

foodborne disease outbreak (FBDO): Defined by the Centers for Disease Control and Prevention (CDC) as an incident in which two or more persons experience a similar illness, and food is implicated.

globalization: The process of increasing the connectivity and interdependence of the world's markets and businesses.

pathogen: A disease-causing microorganism.

zoonosis: A disease that can be transmitted from animals to people or, more specifically, a disease that normally exists in animals but that can infect humans.

Introduction

> *If one recognizes that ensuring food safety*
> *is inherently uncertain, foodborne illnesses become*
> *opportunities to learn rather than failures to predict.*
>
> Porter, et al., 1997

Foodborne disease outbreaks are much more of a concern to the US government and the food industry today than a few decades ago. Many factors have prompted this growing concern (Todd, 1997). First, there have been a growing number of outbreaks associated with food items that were previously considered to be safe. For example, in 1998 there was a large multistate outbreak of *Salmonella* serotype Agona (CDC, 1998). Investigation into the cause of this outbreak implicated toasted oats cereal as the source. Second, foodborne disease outbreaks (FBDOs) have increased in both size and scope over the last decade (Mead, et al., 1999). The impact of these larger FBDOs are an important public health concern due to their impact on children, the aging population, and immunocompromised people. Third, rapid globalization of food production and trade and increased foreign travel have increased the potential likelihood of food contamination. Globalization of the food supply has resulted in the introduction of emerging and reemerging pathogens, many of which are increasingly being associated with the development of life-threatening conditions such as Hemolytic Uremic Syndrome (HUS).

Many foods that were previously considered to be safe from a microbiological point of view are increasingly associated with human infections. Manufactured products, which were once considered to be safe, are increasingly being associated with FBDOs. For example, the 2007 outbreak of *Salmonella* Tennessee infections (more than 400 cases in 44 states) was associated with consumption of peanut butter (CDC, 2007a). There is also an increasing spectrum of fruits and vegetables being associated with FBDOs (Tozzi, Gorietti, & Caprioli, 2001). Contaminated sprouts have caused episodes of salmonellosis and represent an emerging source of *E. coli* O157:H7. Raspberries contaminated with *Cyclospora* have caused several outbreaks in the United States (Herwaldt, 2000). Other fresh produce, such as lettuce, tomatoes, coleslaw, and berries, are established vehicles of Shiga-toxin producing *E. coli* (STEC) infection (Schnirring, 2007; Tozzi, et al., 2001). Unpasteurized fruit juices, increasingly popular among consumers, represent another safety concern. Apple juice, in particular, has been frequently involved in *E. coli* O157:H7 outbreaks (Schnirring, 2007; Tozzi, et al., 2001).

Changes in food production and distribution have had a tremendous affect on the dynamics of FBDOs. Traditional outbreaks typically occurred in limited settings, such as social functions and family gatherings. These outbreaks were usually due to errors in food handling shortly before consumption and were easily recognized by people who were directly involved in the episode and by medical and public health authorities. Today there are an increasing number of large and diffuse outbreaks, involving large geographic areas and even different countries (Tauxe, 2002). These outbreaks are often the result of low-level contamination of widely distributed commercial food items. They are difficult to detect because the increase in cases might not be apparent against the background of sporadic cases. Detection often relies on careful examination of laboratory surveillance data.

These are obvious reasons for the increased concern. According to food safety experts, 2007 was one of the worst years for food safety in US history due to the size and scope of the reported FBDOs. Although it is well accepted that no food safety program is 100% effective, it is obvious that several important issues need to be addressed to prevent, reduce, and control this trend in FBDOs. For example, there are a vast number of entry points created by the inherent qualities of the food system. Susceptibility of livestock and poultry to both pathogenic and commensal microbial agents due to breeding practices and antimicrobial resistance further compound the problems relating to the vast number of entry points inherent in the food system. The ease of worldwide shipment of fresh and frozen foods and the development of new food industries contribute to the increase in size and severity of FBDOs. Finally, the fragmented nature of the food safety system calls into question whether the government can plan more strategically to inspect food production processes, identify and react more quickly to outbreaks of contaminated food, and focus on promoting the safety and integrity of the nation's food supply.

> **Learning Point:** Many foods that were previously considered to be safe from a microbiological point of view are increasingly associated with human infections. Manufactured products, which were once considered to be safe, are increasingly being associated with FBDOs.

Food Safety Begins on the Farm

Many of the microbial agents responsible for FBDOs have a zoonotic origin and have reservoirs in healthy food animals, from which they spread to an increasing variety of foods (Todd, 1997). Microbial pathogens can survive and multiply in animal feed, water troughs, and on the hides of animals, as well as in the intestinal tracts of animals, and they can be passed on through the feces and bodily excretions. Usually, the animal reservoirs are not affected by these pathogens, making them difficult to detect. The trade of infected but apparently healthy animals has facilitated the global spread of many of these zoonotic agents (Nakajima, 1997). Therefore, foods of animal origin are considered to be major vehicles of foodborne infections. While many well-established foodborne pathogens have been controlled or eliminated (e.g., *Mycobacterium bovis* and *Trichinella* spp.) in industrialized countries, many other zoonotic pathogens have been newly described or newly associated with foodborne transmission within the last 25 years, such as *Escherichia coli* O157:H7 in cattle and *Salmonella enteritidis* in layer hens (Tauxe, 2002). Therefore, surveillance must consider the monitoring of healthy animal populations as well as symptomatic animals, and public health concerns must include events that are happening around the world.

Significance of Pathogen Carriage in Livestock, Poultry, and Crops

As mentioned before in a prior chapter, there are several inherent weaknesses in the US agricultural infrastructure. The US agricultural market is highly dependent on large populations of domestic livestock and poultry. These populations are usually bred and reared in close proximity to one another (Chalk, 2004; Cupp, Walker, & Hillison, 2004). The close proximity of farm animals makes them extremely susceptible to infectious agents. The spread of these infectious agents is further compounded by a lack of symptomatic infection in the host animal and the lack of tight regulatory control on the part of the producers. Furthermore, rapid movement of vast amounts of product, including livestock, over broad geographies ensures that pathogenic agents will spread well beyond the original site of a specific outbreak (Chalk, 2004; Cupp, et al., 2004).

Many foodborne pathogens and opportunistic bacteria like enterococci have or can have habitats in food animals (e.g., in the skin and intestinal tract) and can enter meat and milk products during slaughtering and milking, or they can contaminate raw vegetables when the soil is fertilized with untreated manure (Frank, 1997; Busani, Scavia, Luzzi, & Caprioli, 2006). These pathogens can be disseminated to livestock and poultry through a variety of sources. Water is an important vehicle. Water troughs can serve as reservoirs for several pathogenic agents, such as *E. coli* O157:H7 for livestock (LeJune, Besser, & Hancock, 2001). The degree to which water in troughs can serve as a pathogen vehicle can be affected by the presence of rumen content, which influences the survival of various pathogens. Running or standing environmental water, such as rivers, streams, and ponds, can serve as reservoirs of *Campylobacter* spp. (Kemp, et al., 2005). Contaminated feed has been linked to the occurrence of pathogens in livestock and poultry as well (Primm, 1998; Jones, Aitken, Brown, & Collins, 1982). Analyses of commercially manufactured feeds confirmed that both feed ingredients and dust can be sources of *Salmonella* contamination in feed mills (Jones & Richardson, 2004). Moreover, some pathogens, such as *Salmonella* spp., can survive for long periods of time in feed of low water activity (e.g., 16 months at 25°C and 51% relative humidity) (Williams & Benson, 1978). Wildlife and pests can also serve as vehicles for microbial contamination on farms. According to Adhikari, Connolly, Madie, and Davies (2004), indistinguishable isolates of *C. jejuni* have been obtained on the same farm from cattle, flies, and rodents and from the feces of sparrows in a nearby urban area, implying a common source of infection. Studies by Strother, Steelman, and Gbur (2005) illustrate the impact pests can have as vectors of enteric pathogens. They determined that 90% of chickens that consumed a single adult or larval-infected beetle became infected with *Campylobacter*, whereas 100% of birds became *Campylobacter*-positive upon consuming 10 infected beetle adults or larvae.

Vertical transmission of enteric pathogens from parent flocks to progeny has also been demonstrated (Methner, Alshabibi, & Meyer, 1995; Cox, Stern, Hiett, & Berrang, 2002). Semen collection is predisposed to fecal contamination, and subsequent insemination of contaminated material can infect hens and their eggs (Reiber, Conner, & Bilgili, 1995; Donoghue, Blore, Cole, Loskutoff, & Donoghue, 2004). Several antibiotics, including gentamicin, have been effective at reducing bacterial cell numbers without negatively influencing fertility (Sexton, Jacobs, & McDaniel, 1980). Concentrations of antibiotics needed to prevent all bacterial growth, however, were detrimental to fertility (Donoghue, et al., 2004). Antimicrobial dips to sanitize egg surfaces have been used to reduce pathogen contamination of newly hatched chicks. Although single dip treatments of hydrogen peroxide and phenol have proven efficacious in reducing *Salmonella*-positive eggs (Berrang, Cox, Frank, Buhr, & Bailey, 2000), the process usually requires several dips to eliminate *Salmonella* (Cox, et al., 2002).

Animal housing and transportation equipment can harbor pathogens and contribute to contamination of animals; however, a primary source of enteric pathogens transmitted to livestock and poultry is manure. In 1997, it was estimated that 1.36 billion tons of animal manure were produced in the United States, with cattle contributing up to 90% of the burden (US Senate, 1997). The significance of this statistic can be put into perspective by recognizing that five tons of animal manure are produced annually for every living person. Considering this statistic in combination with the high prevalence and high populations of enteric pathogens in animal wastes, it is apparent that manure is a principal source of enteric pathogens on the farm.

Significance of Pathogen Carriage in Crops

Farm ruminants are the major reservoirs for pathogenic contamination of crops. Pathogens, such as *E. coli* O157:H7 are carried asymptomatically and shed transiently in their feces. Both cattle and sheep can excrete high levels of pathogens, leading to significant contamination of the farm environment and pasture. Many bacteria, such as *E. coli* O157:H7, have demonstrated the ability to survive for long periods of time in manure, soil, and pasture runoff. Crops can then be exposed to these environmental pathogens through the application of livestock-composted manure used as fertilizer or irrigation water contaminated with animal feces.

Wildlife and pests have also been implicated as potential vectors of infectious agents, demonstrating a potential alternative when ruminants are not directly present. Pathogens have been isolated from several types of beetles, both adult and larval forms, flies, and from the lesser mealworm. Laboratory experiments have demonstrated that darkling beetles are potential sources of pathogen serotypes of *E. coli* and the lesser mealworms are potential sources of *E. coli, Salmonella,* and *Campylobacter.* Laboratory research has shown that flies can transmit *E. coli* from an environmental source to food products (e.g., the transfer of *E. coli* to apples by fruit flies).

Animal manure represents a significant source of human pathogens. Potential sources of contaminated manure include nearby livestock or poultry operations; nearby municipal wastewater or biosolids storage, treatment, or disposal areas; and high concentrations of wildlife in the growing and harvesting environment (e.g., deer in fields, migratory birds, or bats). Growers should also be alert to the presence of human or animal fecal matter that might be unwittingly introduced into the produce growing and handling environment (e.g., migrant workers). While it is not possible to exclude all animal life from all fresh produce areas, growers can implement practices that reduce the prevalence and likelihood of significant amounts of uncontrolled deposits of animal feces coming into contact with crops (Beuchat & Ryu, 1997).

Irrigation is involved in numerous field operations, including irrigation and application of pesticides and fertilizers, and postharvest operations, such as produce rinsing, cooling, washing, waxing, and transport. The quality of water, how it is used, and the characteristics of the crop influence the potential for water to contaminate produce. The type of crop, the amount of time between contact and harvest, and the postharvest handling practices are important factors. For example, produce that has a large surface area and a rough surface, such as leafy vegetables, foster the entrapment of pathogens and, therefore, present a greater risk than produce with a small smooth surface (FDA, 1998). This is especially true if water contact occurs close to harvest or during postharvest handling. Therefore, it is important that producers consider the source and distribution of the water and its relative potential for being a source of pathogens. They must be aware of the current and historical use of the land and factors such as the following:

1. the prevalence of animal production in the region
2. whether or not feedlots, animal pastures, and dairy operations in the region use fences or other barriers to minimize access to a shared water source
3. whether or not manure is applied to the land by many farms in the region
4. whether or not local rainfall patterns and topography impact the likelihood of contaminated runoff from these operations reaching surface waters
5. whether or not controls are in place to minimize contamination of agricultural waters from other farm or animal operations

These factors all contribute to the potential for microbial contamination and should be identified and controlled by growers to prevent or reduce the incidence of fresh produce contamination.

Among the outbreaks associated with fresh produce consumption with a known etiology, *Salmonella enterica* serotype Enteritidis accounted for the largest number of outbreaks, cases, and deaths (Tauxe, et al., 1997). *E. coli* O157:H7 accounted for the second largest number of outbreaks and was frequently associated with multistate outbreaks. Many pathogens, such as *S. enterica* and *E. coli*, are capable of interacting with the outside surface of plants and fruits and can live in association with other bacteria while obtaining nutrients for their survival (Ji, Smith-Becker, & Keen, 1998).

In recent years, fruits and vegetables, such as cabbage, alfalfa sprouts, tomatoes, and lettuce, have been implicated as vehicles for human infection. These outbreaks are frequently traced back to the growers where a zoonotic source, such as cattle feedlots, deer feces, or other ruminant fecal sources, is identified. For example, numerous outbreaks of salmonellosis had been linked to consumption of contaminated alfalfa sprouts (Stewart, Reineke, Ulaszek, & Tortorello, 2001). These outbreaks have involved a variety of *Salmonella enterica* serotypes, such as Bovismorbificans, Stanley, Newport, Montevideo, Infantalis, Anatum, Tennessee, and Enteritidis. Other alfalfa sprout outbreaks have involved *E. coli* O157:H7 (Como-Sabetti, 1997) and *Bacillus cercus* (Portnoy, Goepfert, & Harmon, 1976). Many of these outbreaks have been traced back to seed contamination (Howard & Hutcheson, 2003). The source of the contamination, in most cases, was indirect contact with animal fecal matter. Because alfalfa sprouts and other seed sprouts are capable of supporting significant microbial populations, sprouts are considered to be an important source of foodborne illness.

> **Learning Point:** Many of the microbial agents responsible for FBDOs have a zoonotic origin and have reservoirs in healthy food animals from which they spread to an increasing variety of foods.

Antimicrobial Resistance

Changes in husbandry practices, such as the nontherapeutic use of antibiotics, contribute to an increase in the stress levels and lower the natural tolerance of animals to disease from contagious organisms (Chalk, 2003). These modifications have also been associated with the development of antimicrobial-resistant bacteria. The emergence of antimicrobial-resistant bacteria has largely been attributed to the widespread use of antibiotics in animal production (Teuber, 2001). Antibiotic resistance develops as a consequence of evolution via natural selection. The antibiotic action is an environmental pressure, and those bacteria that have a mutation that allows them to survive this pressure will live on to reproduce. This trait will then be passed on to their offspring, thereby creating a fully resistant generation. There are several factors that help contribute to the development of antibiotic resistance, such as incorrect diagnosis, unnecessary prescriptions, improper use of antibiotics, and use of antibiotics as livestock feed additives for growth promotion.

Agricultural producers use antibiotics to treat livestock for three primary reasons (NRC, 1998):

1. therapeutically to treat infected animals
2. as a prophylactic to avoid infection of a herd if one animal shows symptoms of an infectious disease
3. as a nutritive at subtherapeutic levels to promote growth

The main infectious diseases that are treated are enteric and pulmonary infections, skin and organ abscesses, and mastitis. The use of antibiotics at subtherapeutic levels for increased growth and feed efficiencies in farm animals, such as pigs, cattle, turkeys, and chickens, is an integral part of modern agriculture worldwide. In the United States, the National Academy of Sciences of America estimated that, in 1978, 6.08 million kilograms of antimicrobials were produced for therapeutic use in agriculture, while 5.58 million kilograms were for addition to animal feed (NAS, 1980). Today it is estimated that greater than 55% of the antibiotics used in the United States are given to food animals in the absence of disease (Mathew, Cissell, & Liamthong, 2007). Nearly 80% of farm animals, mainly cattle, pigs, and poultry, receive subtherapeutic levels of antibiotics in their feed at least part of the time. Although the use of antibiotics in food animal production provides demonstrated benefits, such as improved animal health, higher production, and reduction in foodborne pathogens, bacterial antimicrobial resistance has become a serious problem worldwide (McDermott, et al., 2002).

While overuse and misuse of antibiotics in human medicine contributes greatly to antibiotic resistance, food animal producers use an estimated 70% of all US antibiotics and related drugs nontherapeutically, such as routine feed additive to promote slightly faster growth and to compensate for unsanitary and crowded conditions (Mellon, Benbrook, & Benbrook, 2000; Prescott, 2000). The amount of antibiotics used nontherapeutically in animal agriculture is eight times greater than the amount used in all of human medicine. Furthermore, many of the antibiotics used in animal agriculture are also used in human medicine. The nontherapeutic use of antibiotics involves low-level exposure in feed over long periods of time, which is an ideal method to encourage the development of resistance. In 2002, an Alliance for the Prudent Use of Antibiotics (APUA) analysis of more than 500 scientific articles discovered many lines of evidence linking antimicrobial-resistant human infections to foodborne pathogens of animal origin (APUA, 2002). Resistant human diseases strongly linked to the agricultural overuse of antibiotics include food poisonings caused by *Salmonella* and *Campylobacter*. Antibiotic-resistant bacteria that are commonly transmitted from food animals to people are associated with more infections, longer and more severe illness, more hospitalizations, and an increased fatality rate (Angulo, Nargund, & Chiller, 2004).

Resistant bacteria can be transferred from animals to humans in three ways. First, resistant bacteria can be transferred via food. A study in the Washington, DC area found that 20% of the meat sampled was contaminated with *Salmonella* and that 84% of those bacteria were resistant to antibiotics used in human medicine and animal agriculture (White, et al., 2001). Second, resistant bacteria can be transferred via working with animals. Third, resistant bacteria can be transferred via environmental sources, such as groundwater, surface water, and soil. In most cases, these environmental sources become contaminated through direct contact with animal feces. As mentioned previously, animal feces are a primary source of enteric pathogens. This manure contains resistant bacteria and, thereby, creates an immense pool of resistance genes available for transfer to other bacteria.

According to current research, antibiotic use in food animal production has been associated with the emergence of antibiotic-resistant strains of bacteria including *Salmonella* spp., *Campylobacter* spp., *Escherichia coli*, and *Enterococcus* (Teuber, 1999; Witte, 1998). Fifty years of increasing application of antimicrobial agents has resulted in the enrichment of multiple-antibiotic-resistant bacteria, both pathogenic and commensal, in both human and animal habitats. *Salmonella typhimurium* provides insight into the problem of antibiotic-resistant bacteria. An analysis performed by Huey et al. (1958) indicated that *S. typhimurium* strains isolated from farm animals and humans in the United States between 1940 and 1948 were all sensitive to tetracycline. Following the introduction of tetracycline into human and veterinary medicine, as well as agriculture for growth promotion, the percentage of tetracycline-resistant *S. ty-phimurium* strains has been steadily increasing to more than 90% of the isolated and investigated strains in several countries (Stark, et al., 2006). The usefulness of tetracyclines to fight infectious diseases caused by *S. typhimurium* in farm animals and infected humans was entirely destroyed within 50 years of their first application. *Salmonella* strains from food animals are passed to the human population via insufficiently cooked meat, eggs, and milk (St. Louis, et al., 1988; D'Aoust, 1997). Because enteric infections with *Salmonella* in humans result in multiplication and excretion of the infectious agent in and from the human intestine, the animal-food-human spread must be regarded as an important contribution to the release of antibiotic-resistant bacteria from farm animals. Ceftriaxone-resistant *Salmonella* infections have also been detected in the United States. In one case, infection in a young boy was linked to a strain of *S. typhimurium* variant Copenhagen, acquired from cattle, which was resistant to a total of 13 antibiotics (Fey, et al., 2000). The prevalence of resistance phenotypes in *Salmonella* strains increased from 0.1% in 1996 to 0.5% in 1998, and approximately 77% of the patients affected were younger than 18 years (Dunne, et al., 2000). Finally, multiresistance has become a hallmark of *Salmonella* serotypes such as *S. typhimurium*, *S. Blockley*, and *S. Hadar*.

Research has recently focused on *E. coli* as an indicator species in recent surveillance programs to analyze the antibiotic resistance status of the enteric microflora of both farm animals and humans. In a study by Teuber (2001), 39 isolates out of 50 isolates of Shiga-toxin-producing *E. coli* (STEC) from cattle, ground beef, and humans exhibited resistance to two or more antimicrobial classes, with significant resistance to ampicillin, tetracycline, kanamycin, streptomycin, and sulfamethoxazole. Compared to the overall population, persons with a high level of contact with farm animals have a significant percentage of antibiotic-resistant *E. coli* in their intestinal microflora.

Antimicrobial-resistant *Campylobacter* strains have also been isolated in several studies. For example, Anderson, Yeaton, and Crawford (2001) isolated ciprofloxacin-resistant strains of *Campylobacter jejuni* and *Campylobacter coli* from food of animal origin and from the feces of broilers hens, pigs, and humans. Several of these strains were also found to have a high cross-resistance to nalidixic acid. *C. coli* from pigs had high resistance frequencies to erythromycin (80%) and ampicillin (65%), compared to 34% and 29%, respectively, in humans (Anderson, et al., 2001). *Campylobacter* spp. strains isolated from either human patients or poultry are increasingly resistant to fluoroquinolones since these agents were introduced for use in animals.

Resistant human diseases strongly linked to the agricultural overuse of antibiotics include FBDOs caused by *Salmonella* and *Campylobacter* and postsurgical infections caused by *Enterococcus* (Swartz, 2002). According to Angulo, et al. (2004), an estimated 38 Americans die each day from hospital-acquired antibiotic-resistant infections. Studies have also suggested a link between resistant urinary tract infections caused by *E. coli* and food sources (Manges, et al., 2001). Antibiotic-resistant bacteria that are transmitted from food animals to people are usually associated with more infections, longer and more severe illnesses, more hospitalizations, and an increased fatality rate (Angulo, et al., 2004). Effective antibiotics are essential for the treatment of human illness, especially in children, the elderly, and the immunocompromised.

The substantial evidence from the United States and European Union that these resistant bacteria cause antibiotic-resistant infections in humans has prompted the American Society for Microbiology (ASM), the American Public Health Association (APHA), and the American Medical Association (AMA) to call for substantial restrictions on antibiotic use in food animal production including the end to all nontherapeutic uses. The food animal and pharmaceutical industries have fought hard to prevent new regulations that would limit the use of antibiotics in food animal production. For example, in 2000, the FDA announced their intention to rescind approval for fluoroquinolone use in poultry production because of substantial evidence linking it to the emergence of fluoroquinolone-resistant *Campylobacter* infections in humans. The final decision to ban fluoroquinolones from use in poultry production was not made until five years later due to the challenges from the food animal and pharmaceutical industries.

Since much consideration has been given to the issue of antibiotic use in agriculture on both domestic and international fronts (McDermott, et al., 2002; Who, 1996), many countries have enacted or are considering enacting tighter restrictions on the use of some types of antibiotics in food animal production. Although the ban on the use of growth-promoting antibiotics might result in a decrease in the prevalence of some drug-resistant bacteria, the subsequent increases in animal morbidity and mortality, especially among young animals, might result in higher use of therapeutic antibiotics that often come from drug families of greater relevance to human health. While it is clear that the use of antibiotics can over time result in significant pools of resistance genes among bacteria, the risk posed to humans by resistant organisms from farms and livestock has not been clearly defined. As livestock producers, animal health experts, the medical community, and government agencies consider effective strategies to control overuse and misuse of antibiotics, it is critical that science-based information provide the basis for such considerations. The risks, benefits, and feasibility of such strategies need to be fully considered to maintain both human and animal health while at the same time limiting the risks from antibiotic-resistant bacteria.

> **Learning Point:** Several factors contribute to the development of antibiotic resistance, such as incorrect diagnosis, unnecessary prescriptions, improper use of antibiotics, and use of antibiotics as livestock feed additives for growth promotion.

Globalization of the Food Supply

Over the last few decades, the US food supply has increasingly become more and more global to supply the demand for cheaper food and out of season or exotic food items. According to Gilmore (2004), the United States, like many other countries, is moving from self-sufficiency to an increasing dependence on other countries for its food. However, at the same time, the US regulatory infrastructure for food safety is not adequately prepared and is hindered by an overdependence on the private sector and an underdependence on international cooperation (Gilmore, 2004). Both the FDA and the US Customs and Border Protection agency are not adequately funded nor adequately prepared to ensure the safety of imported food items. The overdependence on the private sector is burdensome for the companies, and it is both insufficient and unreliable to ensure the public's food safety concerns.

Fresh Produce and Globalization

Due to dietary recommendations and campaigns designed to promote health, the overall consumption of fresh produce has increased within the past decade. To meet the growing demand for fresh produce, the amount of produce imported into the United States has increased by more than 250% for fresh vegetables and by more than 155% for fresh fruit since 1980 (Clemens, 2004). At certain times of the year, more than 75% of the fresh fruits and vegetables available in grocery stores and restaurants are imported.

Unfortunately, fresh fruits and vegetables have been responsible for an increasingly larger proportion of FBDOs in the United States. In the last several decades, the proportion of FBDOs associated with produce rose from 0.7% of outbreaks in the 1970s to 6% of outbreaks in the 1990s (Johnston, et al., 2006). Produce-associated outbreaks were also responsible for a higher proportion of all FBDO cases, from 1% (708 of 68,712) of cases in the 1970s to up to 12% (8808 of 74,592) of cases in the 1990s (Sivapalasingam, Friedman, Cohen, & Tauxe, 1997). The increase in incidence of fresh produce-associated FBDOs coincides with the increase in imported fresh produce. According to research, globalization of the food supply is responsible for the introduction of new safety risks and the potential widespread dissemination of contaminated food, particularly produce. For example, consumption of cantaloupes imported from Mexico was associated with multistate outbreaks of *Salmonella enterica* serotype Poona during the spring of consecutive years from 2000 to 2002 (CDC, 2002). Several outbreaks of cyclosporiasis have been traced back to consumption of Guatemalan raspberries, and a 1998 outbreak of *Shigella sonnei* was traced back to consumption of parsley imported from Mexico.

In the United States, the FDA is responsible for the safety of most imported foods, including fresh produce. However, the FDA does not have the legal authority to ensure that international exporters have the proper food production and inspection systems in place. Due to inadequate resources, the FDA inspects only 1% of all foods, including fresh produce, that are imported from other countries. In an effort to improve the safety of imported produce, the FDA published a voluntary guideline in 1998 entitled *Guide to Minimize Microbial Food Safety Hazards for Fresh Fruits and Vegetables* (FDA, 1998). The primary purpose of this guide was to provide the framework for the identification and implementation of practices that are likely to decrease the risk of pathogenic microbiological contamination in produce through the steps of production, packaging, and distribution. The guide is based on both good agricultural practices (GAP) and good manufacturing practices (GMP); however, the guide fails to identify the critical control points at which contamination can occur.

Fish/Seafood and Globalization

The globalization of fish and seafood trade reached $58.2 billion in 2002, an increase of 45% over 1992 levels (Ababouch, 2006). About 38% of the world's fish production enters the international trade market, approximately 50% of which originates in developing countries. The United States, the European Union, and Japan import approximately 80% of the fish traded internationally. With increasing international fish trade and further globalization, there is a greater risk of cross-border transmission of infectious agents (CDC, 2007b). This increase can lead to increased risk to human health and significant implications for international trade. China remains, by far, the largest producer, with reported fish production of 44.3 million metric tons (MMT) in 2002, 16.6 MMT from capture fisheries, and 27.7 MMT from aquaculture. This accounts for approximately 33% (44.4 MMT out of 133.0 MMT worldwide) of the world market.

The most commonly associated pathogens found in fish and seafood include *Vibrio parahaemolyticus, Vibrio vulnificus, Norovirus,* and hepatitis A. The majority of fish and seafood consumed in the United States is imported from countries such as Indonesia, Vietnam, and Thailand, only a small portion of which is inspected. Many fishermen outside of the United States use what is known as the "long-line" fishing method. Using this method, caught fish might be held in water for up to 20 hours before being removed from the line. Bacteria associated with fish and shellfish multiply rapidly if left at ambient temperatures and, thus, can increase the levels of contamination significantly if not rapidly refrigerated after harvest.

Although globalization of the food supply offers many benefits and opportunities, it has also resulted in increased hazards from transboundary foodborne infections (Fidler, 1996). Because food production, manufacturing, and marketing are now global, infectious agents can be disseminated from the original point of processing and packaging to locations thousands of miles away. This multinational approach to food production and distribution and the progressive opening of world markets have allowed the international food trade to flourish while contributing greatly to the increase in size and severity of FBDOs worldwide.

As international trade of food commodities increases, FBDOs of the same origin are more likely to occur in different parts of the globe. Food safety in the late 20th century represents a transitional challenge that requires an enhanced level of international cooperation in the development of standards and regulations as well as enhancement of surveillance systems. Effective food safety programs must be built on a clear understanding of the epidemiology of foodborne diseases throughout the world. Unfortunately, globalization of the world's economy has been accompanied by intense economic competition and increased pressure on governments to downsize, as well as public sector austerity (Berkelman, Bryan, Osterholm, LeDuc, & Hughes, 1994). According to the British Medical Association, these trends might result in a "returning to the 19th century in terms of public health, with problems such as dirty water, contaminated food, and old infectious diseases reemerging" (Ferriman, 1997). Failing a reversal of this trend, public health authorities and health services might be overwhelmed in the near future by outbreaks of foodborne diseases.

Federal Oversight of Surveillance and Regulatory Control

During 2007, consumers were bombarded with reports of food recalls in the media. Outbreaks associated with *E. coli* O157:H7 alone resulted in numerous recalls. For example, a Wisconsin firm recalled more than 800,000 pounds of frozen ground beef patties in October 2007 due to possible *E. coli* O157:H7 contamination (Eamich, 2007; Klein, 2007). In September 2007, a New Jersey-based company recalled more than 21 million pounds of frozen ground beef patties, the fifth largest recall in US history (Hood, 2007). Consumption of the ground beef products, which had been distributed to retail grocery stores and food service institutions throughout the United States, resulted in more than 100 cases of *E. coli* illness in both the United States and Canada. As a result of this recall, the New Jersey-based company, one of the biggest manufacturers of frozen hamburgers in the United States, went out of business. Another recall of ground beef was issued in October 2007 by a company in Florida. According to the USDA's FSIS, the number of *E. coli* recalls climbed to 15 in 2007, compared to five cases in all of 2005.

Salmonella has also been linked to several recalls during 2006 and 2007. For example, Banquet Chicken and Turkey pot pies were removed from the shelves of grocery stores after being linked to at least 139 cases of *Salmonella* in 39 states (CNN, 2006; Earnich, 2007). The same company that made the questionable pot pies also made the peanut butter that had been tainted with *Salmonella* Tennessee that sickened 625 people in 47 states between May 2006 and February 2007 (FDA, 2007b). Recent recalls due to *E. coli* and *Salmonella* have also been linked to fresh produce (CFSAN, 2006; CNN, 2007). For example, *E. coli*-contaminated bagged salad mix and *Salmonella*-contaminated spinach produced in California were among the latest in a string of tainted food reaching the marketplace in 2006, one of the worst years for food safety in US history. In 2006, spinach, also grown in California, was found to be tainted with a particularly virulent form of *E. coli* that sickened more than 200 people and killed three across 26 states (FDA, 2007a).

Marketing surveys have indicated that these recent recalls have had a tremendous affect on consumer confidence (International Food Information Council, 2007; Waldrop, 2007). In a 2007 survey of more than 2000 consumers, only 66% of the respondents expressed confidence that the food they purchased from grocers was safe. This represented a 16-point drop from the confidence levels reported by the Food Policy Institute at Rutgers University a year earlier and was the second-lowest reading in the 18-year history of the poll. Little has occurred to repair the reputation of a food industry that strives to be seen as the world leader in safety. Instead, the news has been highlighted by recalls. According to experts, these problems are just the latest in a long line of mishaps.

Federal Oversight

Like many other federal programs and policies, the food safety system evolved in a piecemeal fashion, typically in response to particular health threats or economic crises (GAO, 2007). The Government Accountability Office (GAO)—the audit, evaluation, and investigative arm of Congress—has designated the federal oversight of food safety as a high-risk area due to its importance to the economy and public health. US agriculture provides an abundant supply of food and other products for Americans and others around the world, annually generating more than $1 trillion in economic activity, including more than $68 billion in exports in 2006. According to the GAO, the federal oversight of food safety is fragmented, resulting in inconsistent oversight, ineffective coordination, and inefficient use of resources. During the past 30 years, the GAO has detailed problems with the current food safety system and has consistently identified several key issues with the current food safety system. Specifically:

- Existing statutes give agencies different regulatory enforcement authorities.
- Federal expenditures on food safety activities are not based on the volume of foods regulated by the agencies.
- Federal agencies are spending resources on overlapping food safety activities.
- Food recalls are voluntary, and federal agencies that are responsible for food safety have no authority to compel companies to carry out recalls.
- There are weaknesses in the flow of critical information among key stakeholders.

According to the GAO, inadequate inspections are just one of a number of problems plaguing the government's food safety system. For example, the FDA inspects companies that grow and process salad greens on average only once every 3 to 9 years, and it inspects only 1% of foods that are imported from other countries. At a time when public confidence in the safety of the food supply is at an all time low, Congress is considering legislation as part of the Farm Bill that would provide potentially weaker safety oversight of the meat industry. The measures would allow small producers that ship their products out of state to forgo the federal inspection program in favor of state inspection programs. Moving to state inspections has the potential to result in more contamination problems if state inspections turn out to be less rigorous, in practice, than the federal meat inspection.

Federal agencies also have difficulties tracing items back to their sources. Tracing a food item back to its source is complicated by several factors. Some companies do not maintain adequate records of food item sources. Many of these companies get food items from distributors who get the items from many sources. For example, any one beef patty can contain meat from several different animals, and one animal can contaminate an entire batch of ground beef. It is not always easy to spot which animals are sick because those carrying potentially harmful pathogens in their intestines usually don't have any symptoms. One of the ways to prevent an asymptomatic animal from entering the food chain is to perform basic microbiological testing on carcasses. However, this can be time consuming and costly. Then there is the larger issue of the industrialization and centralization of the nation's food system. The 2006 spinach recall was for Natural Selection foods. They packed spinach for dozens of different brands. When food supplies are concentrated, small problems can become quite big.

Regulatory Enforcement Authority

The existing statues give different agencies different regulatory oversight and enforcement authority. According to a report by the GAO, there are 15 agencies responsible for the administration of at least 30 laws related to food safety. However, the USDA and FDA have the most responsibility. The USDA is responsible for the safety of meat, poultry, and processed egg products, and the FDA is responsible for virtually all other foods. Among other agencies with responsibilities related to food safety, the National Marine Fisheries Service (NMFS) in the Department of Commerce is responsible for seafood safety and quality; the Environmental Protection Agency (EPA) regulates the use of pesticides and maximum allowable residue levels on food commodities and animal feed; and the Department of Homeland Security (DHS) is responsible for coordinating agencies' food security activities. Furthermore, the GAO has identified 71 interagency agreements that the agencies entered into to better protect public health and to coordinate their food safety efforts. However, the agencies have weak mechanisms for tracking these agreements, which leads to ineffective implementation. Specifically, the FDA and USDA are not fully implementing an agreement to facilitate the exchange of information about dual jurisdiction establishments, which both agencies inspect. In addition, the FDA and NMFS are not implementing an agreement designed to enable each agency to discharge its seafood responsibilities effectively.

The food safety system is further complicated by the subtle differences in food products that dictate which agency regulates a product. For example, which agency is responsible for ensuring the safety of frozen pizzas depends on whether or not meat is used as a topping. If pepperoni or other meats are used as a topping, the manufacturers of the pizzas are inspected by the USDA; otherwise, the FDA inspects manufacturers of frozen cheese or vegetarian pizzas. In other instances, how a food item is packaged determines how it is regulated. For example, regulation of a ham and cheese sandwich depends on how the sandwich is presented. If the sandwich is presented open faced (i.e., only one slice of bread) it is inspected by the USDA, but if presented closed faced (i.e., two slices of bread) it is inspected by the FDA.

Federal Expenditures on Food Safety Activities

Federal expenditures on food safety activities are not based on volume of foods regulated by the agencies. According to the GAO, the majority of federal expenditures for food safety inspection are directed toward the USDA's programs for ensuring the safety of meat, poultry, and egg products. However, the USDA is responsible for regulating only about 20% of the food supply. In contrast, the FDA, which is responsible for regulating about 80% of the food supply, accounted for only 24% of expenditures. Federal funding is made available to support the USDA, which, under current law, is required to maintain continuous inspections at slaughter facilities and examine all slaughtered meat and poultry carcasses. They also visit each processing facility at least once during each operating day. For foods under the FDA's jurisdiction, however, federal law does not mandate the frequency of inspections. According to the FDA, which is responsible for regulating most food products, they do not have enough resources to inspect food processing and distribution facilities on a daily or even monthly basis.

According to the GAO, the overlap in federal food safety oversight also results in misuse of public funding. Federal resources are wasted on a number of overlapping activities, such as inspection/enforcement, training, research, and rule making. For example, both the USDA and FDA conduct similar inspections at 1451 dual jurisdiction establishments, facilities that produce foods regulated by both agencies. Under authority granted by the Bioterrorism Act of

2002, the FDA has the authority to authorize the USDA inspectors to inspect these facilities, but it has not done so. Furthermore, the USDA and FDA maintain separate training programs on similar topics for their inspectors that could be shared.

Surveillance

New and emerging infectious diseases affect humans, domestic animals, livestock, and wildlife and can have significant consequences on health, economics, and biodiversity. Of the emerging infectious diseases of humans, more that 75% are zoonotic. Recent animal health emergencies highlight the vulnerability of the livestock sector to the impact of infectious diseases and the associated risks to human health. Outbreaks have resulted in enormous economic losses globally as well as human illness. Surveillance data on emerging zoonoses are extremely critical in reducing the burden of human, livestock, and wildlife disease. National animal disease emergencies, especially those that affect human health, require a whole-government approach for effective disease containment. Because it is likely that zoonoses and animal diseases with the potential to affect human health will continue to emerge, surveillance and response systems for emerging zoonotic diseases will need to be strengthened and maintained at both national and international levels.

Surveillance of foodborne illness is complicated by several factors (Borgdorff & Motarjemi, 1997). The first is underreporting. Although foodborne illnesses can be severe or even fatal, milder cases are often not detected through routine surveillance. Second, many pathogens transmitted through food are also spread through water or from person to person, thus obscuring the role of foodborne transmission. Finally, some proportion of foodborne illness is caused by pathogens or agents that have not yet been identified and thus cannot be diagnosed. The importance of this final factor cannot be overstated. Many of the pathogens of greatest concern today (e.g., *Campylobacter jejuni, Escherichia coli* O157:H7, *Listeria monocytogenes, Cyclospora cayetanensis*) were not recognized as causes of foodborne illness just 20 years ago.

Federal Recall Authority

Food recall is an important issue, especially in light of recent food recalls, such as the recalls of ground beef, peanut butter, and leafy greens. The primary issue related to food recalls is the discrepancy in the recall authority of the various federal agencies. For example, agencies, such as the National Highway Traffic Safety Administration and the Consumer Product Safety Commission have specific recall authority for many consumer goods that is not available to the USDA or FDA. This includes the authority to (1) require a company to notify the agency when it has distributed a potentially unsafe product; (2) order a recall; (3) establish recall requirements; and (4) impose monetary penalties if a company violates recall requirements. The USDA has no authority to issue mandatory food recall orders, and the FDA's recall authority is limited to infant formula, biological products, medical devices, and radiation-emitting electronic products. The FDA can impose penalties of up to $100,000 per day for a company that fails to recall a defective biological product, such as a vaccine, but it has no authority to penalize a company that is slow to conduct a food recall. Presently, food recalls are largely voluntary.

However, even in the context of their limited recall authority, the GAO (2004) reported that the USDA and FDA could do a better job in carrying out their food recall programs. Specifically, improvements are needed in the data systems used to monitor and manage recalls.

In a report by the GAO in 2003, about 38% and 36% of recalled food was ultimately recovered in recalls overseen by the USDA and FDA, respectively. Furthermore, it was determined that it took USDA staff an average of 38 days to complete verification checks, and the FDA took 31 days. These time frames exceeded the expected shelf life for some of the perishable foods that were recalled, such as fresh ground beef and fresh-cut bagged lettuce. Important dates were not tracked by these agencies, and a lack of adequate funding and understaffing has been consistently listed as the primary reason for these delays.

Industry has also contributed to the delays seen in many recalls. According to the USDA and FDA, there have many instances in which companies were slow to reveal where they had distributed the food or provided inaccurate customer lists. Distribution information is critical during food recalls. The USDA and FDA uses this information to monitor the effectiveness of a company's recall actions by contacting a sample of the distribution chain from these lists to verify that retail customers have received notice of the recall and located and removed the food item from the marketplace. In recent years, the volume of food that companies recalled in the United States substantially increased, making this an important part of the response. For example, in 1988 the meat and poultry industries recalled nearly 6 million pounds of product, while in 2003, the meat and poultry industries recalled nearly 36 million pounds of product.

These weaknesses heighten the risk that unsafe food will remain in the food supply and ultimately be consumed and is underscored in the recent outbreaks of *Escherichia coli* O157:H7 in spinach and *Salmonella* in peanut butter, along with the outbreaks of contaminated pet food.

Learning Point: Both the FDA and the Customs and Border Protection agency are not adequately funded nor adequately prepared to ensure the safety of imported food items. The overdependence on the private sector is burdensome for companies, and it is both insufficient and unreliable to ensure the public's food safety concerns.

Chapter Summary

Despite reassurances from federal and state officials that the American food supply is among the safest in the world, there is growing concern about the occurrence of both naturally occurring foodborne disease outbreaks and bioterrorism. This concern is supported by foodborne disease outbreak statistics published annually by the CDC, which states that there are approximately 76 million cases of foodborne illnesses in the United States each year, about 325,000 of which require hospitalization and about 5000 of which result in death. Media attention of recent outbreaks of *E. coli* O157:H7 in spinach and *Salmonella* in peanut butter highlight the risks posed by accidental food contamination. Industry representatives estimated that losses from the recent California spinach *E. coli* outbreak ranged from $37 million to $74 million. The attacks of 9/11 heightened awareness that the food supply could also be vulnerable to deliberate contamination. According to Gilmore (2004), when it comes to the prospect of an attack against crops, livestock, poultry, and fish using biological agents, the United States has rolled out the welcome mat (Gilmore, 2004). According to former Agriculture Secretary Dan Glickman, the system in place today to protect the agriculture and food infrastructures is poorly suited to modern threats.

Recent outbreaks add fuel to a fiery debate over the effectiveness of the nation's food safety network. Critics contend that the network is outdated, understaffed, and often lacks the necessary momentum to demand the performance from companies that the public expects. Critics argue that although many facets of food safety have improved, such as surveillance, many weaknesses remain. They suggest that lawmakers act decisively and immediately to give the FDA, USDA, and relevant state agencies mandatory recall authority to remove tainted food from the marketplace. Furthermore, Congress should establish a single food safety agency to ensure better safety of our nation's food supply, with substantial resources to hire more inspectors and enforce good agricultural practices (GAP) and hazard analysis critical control point (HACCP) programs at every farm and every processing facility. GAP and HACCP are generally recognized food safety procedures and principles developed by academia, industry, or government that are not universally enforced. According to these critics, until the highest safety standards are rigorously enforced by a single agency that has robust, mandatory authority to inspect food, farms, and processors and to recall contaminated foods from the marketplace, consumers should not stop worrying about the safety of their meal. Finally, because prevention of foodborne diseases is a multifactorial process, an understanding of the mechanisms by which contamination occurs along the chain of food production and the ways that infections can be transmitted to humans is necessary for any prevention strategy.

Issues to Debate

1. How could we change the food system (i.e., the structure) to make it safer?
2. Can pathogen carriage be reduced in livestock and crops, and if so, how?
3. How can genetic engineering improve food safety (think in terms of antibiotic and pesticide resistance)?
4. What steps can the government take to improve food safety oversight?
5. What role does industry and the consumer play in improving federal oversight?

References

Ababouch, L. (2006). Assuring fish safety and quality in international fish trade. *Marine Pollution Bulletin, 53,* 561–568.

Adhikari, B. J., Connolly, J. H., Madie, P., & Davies, P. R. (2004). Prevalence and clonal diversity of *Campylobacter jejuni* from dairy farms and urban sources. *New Zealand Veterinary Journal, 52,* 378–383.

Anderson, S. A., Yeaton, W., & Crawford, L. M. (2001). Risk assessment of the impact on human health of resistant *Campylobacter jejuni* from fluoroquinolone use in beef cattle. *Food Control, 12,* 13–25.

Angulo, F. J., Nargund, V. N., & Chiller, T. C. (2004). Evidence of an association between use of antimicrobial agents in food animals and antimicrobial resistance among bacteria isolated from humans and the human consequences of such resistance. *Journal of Veterinary Medicine, 51,* 374–379.

APUA. (2002). *From farm to fork: Scientific alliance calls for more stringent policy on antibiotic use in agriculture.* Retrieved October 13, 2007, from http://www.tufts.edu

Berkelman, R. L., Bryan, R. T., Osterholm, M. T., LeDuc, J. W., & Hughes, J. M. (1994). Infectious disease surveillance: A crumbling foundation. *Science, 264,* 368–370.

Berrang, M. E., Cox, N. A., Frank, J. F., Buhr, R. J., & Bailey, J. S. (2000). Hatching egg sanitization for prevention or reduction of human enteropathogens. *Journal of Applied Poultry Research, 9,* 279–284.

Beuchat, L. R., & Ryu, J. H. (1997). Produce handling and processing practices. *Emerging Infectious Diseases, 3,* 459–465.

Borgdorff, M. W., & Motarjemi, Y. (1997). Foodborne disease surveillance: What are the options? *World Health Statistics Quarterly, 50,* 12–23.

Breithaupt, G. (2005). Large animal vets are on the decline in rural areas. *Mount Vernon News.* Retrieved October 10, 2007, from http://www.mountvernonnews.com

Busani, L., Scavia, G., Luzzi, I., & Caprioli, A. (2006). Laboratory surveillance for prevention and control of foodborne zoonoses. *Annali Dell Istituto Superiore Di Sanita, 42,* 401–404.

Centers for Disease Control and Prevention. (1998). Multistate outbreak of *Salmonella* serotype Agona infections linked to toasted oats cereal, United States, April–May, 1998. *Morbidity and Mortality Weekly Report, 47,* 462–464.

Centers for Disease Control and Prevention. (2002). Multistate outbreaks of *Salmonella* serotype Poona infections associated with eating cantaloupe from Mexico—United States and Canada, 2000-2002. *Morbidity and Mortality Review, 51,* 1044–1047.

Centers for Disease Control and Prevention. (2007a). Multistate outbreak of *Salmonella* serotype Tennessee infections associated with peanut butter—United States, 2006-2007. *Morbidity and Mortality Weekly Report, 56,* 521–524.

Centers for Disease Control and Prevention. (2007b). Scombroid fish poisoning associated with tuna steaks—Louisiana and Tennessee, 2006. *Morbidity and Mortality Weekly Report, 56,* 817–819.

Centers for Food Safety and Applied Nutrition. (2006). *Nationwide E. coli O157:H7 outbreaks.* Retrieved October 12, 2007, from http://www.cfsan.fda.gov

Chalk, P. (2003). *The bioterrorist threat to agricultural livestock and produce* (Testimony before the US Senate). Retrieved October 10, 2007, from http://www.rand.org

Chalk, P. (2004). *Hitting America's soft underbelly: The potential threat of deliberate biological attack against the US agricultural and food industry.* Retrieved October 10, 2007, from http://www.rand.org

Clemens, R. (2004). *The expanding US market for fresh produce.* Center for Agriculture and Rural Development. Retrieved October 15, 2007, from http://www.agmrc.org

CNN. (2007). *Frozen pot pies suspected in* Salmonella *outbreak.* Retrieved October 12, 2007, from http://www.cnn.com

CNN. (2007). *E. coli outbreak linked to California spinach field.* Retrieved October 12, 2007, from http://www.cnn.com

Como-Sabetti, K. (1997). Outbreaks of *E. coli* O157:H7 infection associated with eating alfalfa sprouts Michigan and Virginia, June–July 1997. *Morbidity and Mortality Weekly Report, 46,* 741–745.

Cox, N. A., Stern, N. J., Hiett, K. L., & Berrang, M. E. (2002). Identification of a new source of *Campylobacter* contamination in poultry: Transmission from breeder hens to broiler chickens. *Avian Diseases, 46,* 535–541.

Cupp, O.S., Walker, D. E., & Hillison, J. (2004). Agroterrorism in the US: Key security challenges for the 21st century. *Biosecurity and Bioterrorism, 2,* 97–105.

D'Aoust, J. Y. (1997). *Salmonella* species. In M.P. Doyle, L.R. Beuchat, & T. Montville (Eds.), *Food microbiology—Fundamentals and frontiers* (pp. 129–158). Washington, DC: ASM.

Donoghue, A. M., Blore, P. J., Cole, K., Loskutoff, N. M., & Donoghue, D. J. (2004). Detection of *Campylobacter* or *Salmonella* in turkey semen and the ability of poultry semen extenders to reduce their concentrations. *Poultry Science, 83,* 1728–1733.

Dunne, E. F., Fey, P. D., Kludt, P., Reporter, R., Mostashari, F., Shillam, P., et. al. (2000). Emergence of domestically-acquired ceftriaxone-resistant *Salmonella* infections associated with AmpC β-lactamase. *Journal of the American Medical Association, 284,* 3151–3156.

Earnich, A. (2007). Missouri firm recalls frozen pot pie products for possible *Salmonella* contamination. Retrieved October 15, 2007, from http://www.fsis.usda.gov

FAO. (1996). *The World Food Summit* (FAO Technical Background Document Number 12).

Ferriman, A. (1997). Doctors warn of a return of past plagues. *The Independent.*

Fey, P. D., Safranek, T. J., Rupp, M. E., Dunne, E. F., Ribot, E., Iwen, P. C., et al. (2000). Ceftriaxone-resistant *Salmonella* infection acquired by a child from cattle. *New England Journal of Medicine, 342,* 1242–1249.

Fidler, D. (1996). Globalization, international law and emerging infectious diseases. *Emerging Infectious Diseases, 2,* 77–84.

Food and Drug Administration. (1998). *Guide for industry: Guide to minimize microbial food safety hazards for fresh fruits and vegetables.* Retrieved October 15, 2007, from http://vm.cfsan.fda.gov/~dms/proddrf2.html

Food and Drug Administration. (2007a). FDA finalizes report on 2006 spinach outbreak. Retrieved October 5, 2007, from http://www.fda.gov

Food and Drug Administration. (2007b). Update on *Salmonella* outbreak and Peter Pan peanut butter and Great Value peanut butter. Retrieved October 5, 2007, from http://www.fda.gov

Frank, J. F. (1997). Milk and dairy products. In M. P. Doyle, L. R. Beuchat, & T. J. Montville (Eds.), *Food microbiology—fundamentals and frontiers* (pp. 101–116). Washington, DC: ASM.

GAO. (2004). *Food safety: USDA and FDA need to better ensure prompt and complete recalls of potentially unsafe food* (Report to Congressional requesters). Retrieved September 14, 2007, from http://www.gao.gov/new.items/d0551.pdf

GAO. (2007). *Federal oversight of food safety: High-risk designation can bring attention to limitations in the government's food recall program* (Testimony before the Subcommittee on Oversight and Investigations, Committee on Energy and Commerce, House of Representatives). Retrieved September 10, 2007, from http://www.gao.gov/new.items/d07785t.pdf

Gilmore, R. (2004). US food safety under siege? *Nature Biotechnology, 22,* 1503–1505.

Gregory, P. J., Ingram, J. S., & Brklacich, M. (2005). Climate change and food security. *Philosophical Transactions of the Royal Society, 360,* 2139–2148.

Herwaldt, B. L. (2000). *Cyclospora cayetanensis*: A review, focusing on the outbreaks of cyclosporiasis in the 1990s. *Clinical Infectious Diseases, 31,* 1040–1057.

Hood, S. R. (2007). *Topps E. coli beef recall linked to tainted Canadian beef.* Retrieved October 29, 2007, from http://rockhill.injuryboard.com

Howard, M. B., & Hutcheson, S. W. (2003). Growth dynamics of *Salmonella enteric* strains on alfalfa sprouts and in waste seed irrigation water. *Applied and Environmental Microbiology, 69,* 548–553.

Huey, C. R. & Edwards, P. R. (1958). Resistance of *Salmonella typhimurium* to tetracyclines. *Proceedings of the Society for Experimental Biology and Medicine, 97,* 550–551.

International Food Information Council. (2007). *Food biotechnology: A study of US consumer attitudinal trends, 2007 report.* Retrieved October 12, 2007, from http://www.ific.org

Ji., C., Smith-Becker, J., & Keen, N. T. (1998). Genetics of plant-pathogen interactions. *Current Opinions in Biotechnology, 9,* 202–207.

Johnston, L. M., Jaykus, L. A., Moll, D., Ancisco, J., Mora, B., & Moe, C. L. (2006). A field study of the microbiological quality of fresh produce of domestic and Mexican origin. *International Journal of Food Microbiology, 112,* 83–95.

Jones, F. T., & Richardson, K. E. (2004). *Salmonella* in commercially manu-factured feeds. *Poultry Science, 83,* 384–391.

Jones, P. W., Aitken, M., Brown, G. T. H., & Collins, P. (1982). Transmission of *Salmonella* mbandaka to cattle from contaminated feed. *Journal of Hygiene, 88,* 255–263.

Kemp, R. A., Leatherbarrow, J. H., Williams, N. J., Hart, C. A., Clough, H. E., Turner, J., et al. (2005). Prevalence and genetic diversity of *Campylobacter* spp. in environmental water samples from a 100-square-kilometer predominantly dairy farming area. *Applied Environmental Microbiology, 71,* 1876–1882.

Klein, M. (2007). *Cargill Meat Solutions recalls frozen ground beef patties.* Retrieved October 10, 2007, from http://www.cargill.com

LeJeune, J. T., Besser, T. E., & Hancock, D. D. (2001). Cattle water troughs as reservoirs of *Escherichia coli* O157. *Applied Environmental Microbiology, 67,* 3053–3057.

Manges, A. R., Johnson, J. R., Foxman, B., O'Bryan, T. T., Fullerton, K.E., & Riley, L. W. (2001). Widespread distribution of urinary tract infections caused by a multidrug-resistant *Escherichia coli* clonal group. *New England Journal of Medicine, 345,* 1007–1013.

Mathew, A. G., Cissell, R., & Liamthong, S. (2007). Antibiotic resistance in bacteria associated with food animals: A United States perspective of livestock production. *Foodborne Pathogens and Disease, 4,* 115–133.

McDermott, P. E., Zhao, S., Wagner, D. D., Simjee, S., Walker, R. D., & White, D. G. (2002). The food safety perspective of antibiotic resistance. *Animal Biotechnology, 13,* 71–84.

Mead, P. S., Slutsker, L., Dietz, V., McCaig, L. F., Bresee, J. S., Shapiro, C., et al. (1999). Food-related illness and death in the United States. *Emerging Infectious Diseases, 5,* 607–625.

Mellon, M., Benbrook, C., & Benbrook, K. (2000). *Hogging it: Estimates of antimicrobial abuse in livestock.* Retrieved October 12, 2007, from http://www.ucsusa.org

Methner, U., Alshabibi, S., & Meyer, H. (1995). Experimental oral infection of specific pathogen-free laying hens and cocks with *Salmonella enteritidis* strains. *Journal of the Veterinary Medical Service, 42,* 459–469.

Nakajima, H. (1997). Global disease threats and foreign policy. *Brown Journal of World Affairs.*

National Academy of Sciences. (1980). *The effects on human health of subtherapeutic use of antimicrobials in animal feeds.* Washington, DC: Author.

National Research Council & Institute of Medicine. (1998). *The use of drugs in food animals: Benefits and risks.* Washington, DC: National Academy Press.

Portnoy, B., Goepfert, J., & Harmon, S. (1976). An outbreak of *B. cereus* food poisoning resulting from contaminated vegetable sprouts. *American Journal of Epidemiology, 10,* 589–594.

Potter, M., Gonzalez-Ayala, S., & Silarug, N. (1997). The epidemiology of foodborne diseases. In M. P. Doyle, L. Beuchat, T. Montville, (Eds).

Fundamentals of Food Microbiology. Washington, (DC): American Society for Microbiology.

Prescott, J. F. (2000). Antimicrobial drug resistance and its epidemiology. In J. F. Prescott, J. D. Baggot, & R. D. Walker (Eds.), *Antimicrobial therapy in veterinary medicine* (3rd ed.) (pp. 27–49). Ames, IA: Iowa State University Press.

Primm, N. D. (1998). Field experience with the control of salmonellae introduction into turkey flocks via contaminated feeds. *Proceedings of the Western Poultry Disease Conference, 47,* 27–29.

Reiber, M. A., Conner, D. E., & Bilgili, S. F. (1995). *Salmonella* colonization and shedding patterns of hens inoculated via semen. *Avian Diseases, 39,* 317–322.

Sexton, T. J., Jacobs, L. A., & McDaniel, G. R. (1980). New poultry semen extender: Effect of antibacterials in control of bacterial contamination in chicken semen. *Poultry Science, 59,* 274–281.

Schnirring, L. (2007). CDC says some foodborne illnesses rose in 2006. Retrieved October 10, 2007, from http://www.cidrap.umn.edu

Sivapalasingam, S., Friedman, C. R., Cohen, L., & Tauxe, R. V. (1997). Fresh produce: A growing cause of outbreaks of foodborne disease in the United States, 1973 through 1997. *Journal of Food Protection, 67,* 2342–2353.

St. Louis, M. E., Morse, D. L., Potter, M. E., DeMelfi, T. M., Guzewich, J. J., & Tauxe, R. V. (1988). The emergence of Grade A eggs as a major source of *Salmonella enteritidis* infections: Implications for the control of salmonellosis. *Journal of the American Medical Association, 259,* 2103–2107.

Stark, K., Regula, G., Hernandez, J., Knopf, L., Fuchs, K., Morris, R. S., et al. (2006). Concepts for risk-based surveillance in the field of veterinary medicine and veterinary public health: Review of current approaches. *BioMed Central Health Services Research, 6,* 20–28.

Stewart, D., Reineke, K., Ulaszek, J., & Tortorello, M. (2001). Growth of *Salmonella* during sprouting of alfalfa seeds associated with salmonellosis outbreaks. *Journal of Food Protection, 64,* 618–622.

Strother, K. O., Steelman, C. D., & Gbur, E. E. (2005). Reservoir competence of lesser mealworm (Coleoptera: Tenebrionidae) for *Campylobacter jejuni* (Campylobacterales: Campylobacteraceae). *Journal of Medical Entomology, 42,* 42–47.

Swartz, M. (2002). Human diseases caused by foodborne pathogens of animal origin. *Clinical Infectious Diseases, 34,* S111–S122.

Tauxe, R. V. (2002). Emerging foodborne pathogens. *International Journal of Food Microbiology, 78,* 31–41.

Tauxe, R., Kruse, H., Hedberg, C., Potter, M., Madden, J., & Wachsmuth, K. (1997). Microbial hazards and emerging issues associated with produce: A preliminary report to the National Advisory Committee on Microbiologic Criteria for Foods. *Journal of Food Protection, 60,* 1400–1408.

Teuber, M. (1999). Spread of antibiotic resistance with foodborne pathogens. *Cellular and Molecular Life Sciences, 56,* 755–763.

Teuber, M. (2001). Veterinary use and antibiotic resistance. *Current Opinions in Microbiology, 4,* 493–499.

Todd, E. C. (1997). Epidemiology of foodborne diseases. *A Worldwide Review, 50,* 30–50.

Tozzi, A. E., Gorietti, S., & Caprioli, A. (2001). Epidemiology of human infections by *Escherichia coli* O157 and other verocytotoxin-producing *E. coli.* In G. Duffy, P. Garvey, & D. McDowell (Eds.), *Verocytotoxigenic Escherichia coli* (pp. 161–179). Trumbull, CT: Food & Nutrition Press.

US Senate Agriculture Committee, Democratic Staff. (1997). *Animal waste pollution in America: An emerging national problem* (Report compiled by the Minority Staff of the United States Senate Committee on Agriculture, Nutrition, and Forestry for Senator Tom Harkin [D-IA]). Retrieved October 10, 2007, from http://www.senate.gov/~agriculture/animalw.htm

Waldrop, C. (2007). Consumer Federation of America Docket number 2007N-0051. Retrieved October 10, 2007, from http://www.consumerfed.org

White, D. G., Zhao, S., Sudler, R., Ayers, S., Friedman, S., Chen, S., et al. (2001). The isolation of antibiotic-resistant *Salmonella* from retail ground meats. *New England Journal of Medicine, 345,* 1147–1154.

Williams, J. E., & Benson, S. T. (1978). Survival of *Salmonella* Typhimurium in poultry feed and litter at three temperatures. *Avian Diseases, 22,* 742–747.

Witte, W. (1998). Medical consequences of antibiotic use in agriculture. *Science, 279,* 996–997.

WHO. (1996). *International response to epidemics and applications of the international health regulations* (Report of a WHO consultation). Geneva, Switzerland: Author.

CHAPTER 12

PRINCIPLES AND APPLICATION OF THE HAZARD ANALYSIS AND CRITICAL CONTROL POINTS

Tamara M. Crutchley Bushell, PhD

Chapter Objectives

After reading the chapter and reflecting on the contents, you should be able to:

1. Explain the importance of the HACCP process control system.
2. Understand the differences between traditional food safety systems and the HACCP process control system.
3. Identify the seven principles of the HACCP process control system.
4. Describe the logical sequence for application of the HACCP system.
5. Understand the use of HACCP in the various food industries.

Key Terms

critical control point (CCP): A step at which control can be applied and is essential to prevent or eliminate a food safety hazard or reduce it to an acceptable level.

critical limit: A criterion that separates acceptability from unacceptability.

deviation: Failure to meet a critical limit.

flow diagram: A systematic representation of the sequence of steps or operations used in the production or manufacture of a particular food item.

HACCP: A system that identifies, evaluates, and controls hazards that are significant for food safety.

HACCP plan: A document prepared in accordance with the principles of HACCP to ensure control of hazards that are significant for food safety in the segment of the food chain under consideration.

hazard: A biological, chemical, or physical agent in, or condition of, food with the potential to cause an adverse health effect.

hazard analysis: The process of collecting and evaluating information about hazards and conditions that lead to the presence to decide which are significant for food safety and therefore should be addressed in the HACCP plan.

monitor: The act of conducting a planned sequence of observations or measurements of control parameters to assess whether a CCP is under control.

step: A point, procedure, operation, or stage in the food chain, including raw materials, from primary production to final consumption.

validation: Obtaining evidence that the elements of the HACCP plan are effective.

verification: The application of methods, procedures, tests, and other evaluations, in addition to monitoring, to determine compliance with the HACCP plan.

Introduction

The food safety system, which developed early in the 20th century, was largely based on organoleptic (sight, touch, and smell) methods (FDA, 2001b). Traditional regulatory methods for food safety were based on observation and testing of samples, as well as detection of spoilage. These methods were relatively sufficient during the early part of the 20th century because the major public health concerns of the time were the potential for transmission of diseases from sick animals to humans and the lack of sanitary conditions for animal slaughter and production of processed products. However, this system has changed little over time and, due to increases in supply and demand, it is no longer effective.

The HACCP system was developed in 1959 by the Pillsbury Company in collaboration with the US National Aeronautics and Space

Administration (NASA) as a means to ensure food safety for the first manned space mission. Limitations of traditional end product testing became evident to those who were trying to provide the safest food products. To ensure that the food used for the space mission would be safe, almost all of the manufactured product was used during the testing, leaving very little for actual use. The proactive system of HACCP evolved from these efforts to understand and control food safety failures.

The HACCP system is a scientific approach to process control. Unlike traditional approaches, which use organoleptic methods for identifying contamination of end products, HACCP uses control measures to prevent or reduce contamination during processing through the use of steps that are designed to address physical, chemical, and biological hazards and by addressing deviations as soon as they are detected. The HACCP system can be used at all stages of food production and offers a number of advantages over the traditional food safety system. Most importantly, HACCP

- focuses on identifying and preventing hazards from contaminating foods
- is based on sound science
- permits more efficient and effective government oversight, primarily because the record keeping allows investigators to see how well a firm complys with food safety laws over a period rather than how well it is doing on any given day
- places the responsibility for ensuring food safety appropriately on the food manufacturer or distributor
- helps food companies compete more effectively in the world market
- reduces barriers to international trade

Since the mid-1970s, HACCP has been widely used by industry and government, and today it is recognized both nationally and internationally as a logical tool for adapting traditional inspection methods to a modern, science-based food safety system. The HACCP system was designed to identify specific hazards and measures for controlling contamination and can be applied throughout the food chain from primary production to final consumption. Its successful application, however, requires the full commitment and involvement of management and the workforce. It also requires a multidisciplinary approach, which includes the expertise of agronomy, veterinary health, production, microbiology, medicine, public health, food technology, environmental health, chemistry, and engineering.

The Seven HACCP Principles

The HACCP process control system is based on the seven principles that were articulated by the National Advisory Committee on Microbiological Criteria for Foods (NACMCF) in 1992. The NACMCF, which was established in 1988, provides impartial, scientific advice to federal food safety agencies for use in the development of an integrated national food safety system approach from farm to final consumption to assure the safety of domestic, imported, and exported foods (USDA, 2007). In 1995, the NACMCF revised their 1992 principles to coincide with information and guidelines obtained from the Codex Committee on Food Hygiene. The following are the revised HACCP principles:

Principle 1: *Conduct a hazard analysis.*

- Potential hazards associated with a food and measures to control those hazards are identified.
- These hazards can be biological, such as a microbe; chemical, such as a toxin; or physical, such as ground glass or metal fragments.
- Plants determine the food safety hazards and identify the preventive measures that they can apply to control these hazards.
- These are risks associated with growing, harvesting, processing, distributing, preparing, and/or using raw material or food products.
- Hazard usually means the contamination, growth, or survival of microorganisms related to food safety or spoilage.
- A hazard can also include dangerous chemical contaminants or foreign objects (glass or metal fragments).
- Risk is the estimate of how likely it is that the hazard will occur.

Principle 2: *Identify critical control points.*

- These are points in a food's production—from its raw state through processing and shipping to consumption by the consumer—at which the potential hazard can be controlled or eliminated. Examples are cooking, cooling, packaging, and metal detection.

- A critical control point (CCP) is a point, step, or procedure in a food process at which control can be applied and, as a result, a food safety hazard can be prevented, eliminated, or reduced to an acceptable level. A food safety hazard is any *biological, chemical,* or *physical* property that can cause a food to be unsafe for human consumption.
- The effectiveness of control at CCP depends on the correct identification of a hazard, the appropriateness of the CCP, the adequacy of control measures, the correctness of critical limits, the capability of monitoring methods to detect deviations from normality in time, the appropriateness of monitoring frequency, and the adequacy of process control adjustments.
- A critical control point is a location, practice, procedure, or process that can be used to minimize or prevent unacceptable contamination, survival, or growth of foodborne pathogens or spoilage organisms or the introduction of unwanted chemicals or foreign objects.

Principle 3: *Establish critical limits for each critical control point.*

- A *critical limit* is the maximum or minimum value to which a physical, biological, or chemical hazard must be controlled at a critical control point to prevent, eliminate, or reduce the hazard to an acceptable level.
- For a cooked food, for example, this might include setting the minimum cooking temperature and time required to ensure the elimination of any harmful microbes.
- Monitoring systems must be able to effectively determine if a CCP is under control.
- Corrective action must be defined to be used when a CCP monitoring point shows that the system is out of control.

Principle 4: *Establish critical control point monitoring requirements.*

- Monitoring activities are necessary to ensure that the process is under control at each critical control point. FSIS requires that each monitoring procedure and its frequency be listed in the HACCP plan.

- Such procedures might include determining how and by whom cooking time and temperature should be monitored.

Principle 5: *Establish corrective actions.*

- These are actions to be taken when monitoring indicates a deviation from an established critical limit. The final rule requires a plant's HACCP plan to identify the corrective actions to be taken if a critical limit is not met. Corrective actions are intended to ensure that no product that is injurious to health or otherwise adulterated as a result of the deviation enters commerce.
- For example, food should be reprocessed or disposed of if the minimum cooking temperature is not met.

Principle 6: *Establish record keeping procedures.*

- The HACCP regulation requires that all plants maintain certain documents, including their hazard analysis and written HACCP plan, and record the monitoring of critical control points, critical limits, verification activities, and the handling of processing deviations.
- For example, time- and temperature-recording devices are tested to verify that a cooking unit is working properly.

Principle 7: *Establish procedures for verifying that the HACCP system is working as intended.*

- *Validation* ensures that the plans do what they were designed to do, that is, they are successful in ensuring the production of safe product. Plants will be required to validate their own HACCP plans. FSIS will not approve HACCP plans in advance, but it will review them for conformance with the final rule.
- *Verification* ensures that the HACCP plan is adequate, that is, it works as intended. Verification procedures can include such activities as review of HACCP plans, CCP records, critical limits, and microbial sampling and analysis. FSIS is requiring that the HACCP plan includes verification tasks to be performed by plant personnel. Verification tasks would also be performed by FSIS inspectors. Both FSIS and industry will undertake microbial testing as one of several verification activities.

- This would include records of hazards and their control methods, the monitoring of safety requirements, and action taken to correct potential problems.

> **Learning Point:** Each of these principles must be backed by sound scientific knowledge, for example, published microbiological studies on time and temperature factors for controlling foodborne pathogens.

Guidelines for the Application of the HACCP System

Prior to application of HACCP to any sector of the food chain, each sector should be built on a solid foundation of prerequisite programs (FDA, 2001b). To protect food while under its control, segments of the food industry have traditionally used programs such as good manufacturing practices (GMP). These conditions and practices are now considered to be prerequisites for the development and implementation of effective HACCP plans. Some of the common prerequisite conditions and practices include the following:

- The establishment should be located, constructed, and maintained according to sanitary design principles, with a linear product flow and traffic control to minimize cross-contamination from raw to cooked materials.
- Each facility should assure that its suppliers have effective GMP and food safety programs in place.
- There should be written specifications for all ingredients, products, and packaging materials.
- All equipment should be constructed and installed according to sanitary design principles and should include documented preventive maintenance and calibration schedules.
- All procedures for cleaning and sanitation of the equipment and the facility should be written and followed.
- All employees and other persons who enter the manufacturing plant should follow the requirements for personal hygiene.
- All employees should receive documented training in personal hygiene, GMP, cleaning and sanitation procedures, personal safety, and their role in the HACCP program.

- Documented procedures must be in place to assure the segregation and proper use of nonfood chemicals in the plant, including cleaning chemicals, fumigants, and pesticides or baits used in or around the plant.
- All raw materials and products should be stored under sanitary conditions and the proper environmental conditions, such as temperature and humidity, to assure their safety and wholesomeness.
- All raw materials and products should be lot coded, and a recall system should be in place, so that rapid and complete traces and recalls can be done when a product retrieval is necessary.
- Effective pest control programs should be in place.

Logic Sequence for Application of HACCP

According to the FAO/WHO (1998), the application of the seven HACCP principles consists of the following tasks as identified in the Logic Sequence for Application of HACCP.

1. *Assemble HACCP team*
   To ensure that the appropriate product-specific knowledge and expertise is available for the development of an HACCP plan, a multidisciplinary team should be assembled. Where such expertise is not available on site, expert advice should be obtained from other sources. The scope of the HACCP plan should be identified and should describe the segment of the food chain involved and the general classes of hazards to be addressed (e.g., does it cover all classes of hazards or only selected classes?).
2. *Describe product*
   A full description of the product, which includes the relevant safety information (i.e., composition, physical/chemical structure, microcidal/static treatment, packaging, durability, storage conditions, methods of distribution, etc.), should be drawn up.
3. *Identify intended use*
   The intended use should be based on the expected uses of the product by the end user or consumer, including considerations regarding vulnerable groups of the population (e.g., children, pregnant women, the elderly, and the immunocompromised).

FIGURE 12.1   Logic Sequence for the Application of HACCP

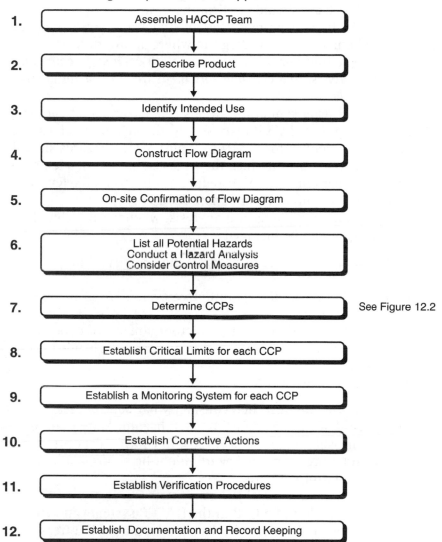

1. Assemble HACCP Team

2. Describe Product

3. Identify Intended Use

4. Construct Flow Diagram

5. On-site Confirmation of Flow Diagram

6. List all Potential Hazards
   Conduct a Hazard Analysis
   Consider Control Measures

7. Determine CCPs   See Figure 12.2

8. Establish Critical Limits for each CCP

9. Establish a Monitoring System for each CCP

10. Establish Corrective Actions

11. Establish Verification Procedures

12. Establish Documentation and Record Keeping

Source: World Health Organization. Retrieved December 27, 2007, from http://www.who.int/foodsafety/fs_management/en/intro_haccp_figures.pdf.

4. *Construct flow diagram*

A flow diagram, which covers all steps in the operation, should be constructed by the HACCP team, taking into consideration both the steps preceding and following the specified operation.

5. *On-site confirmation of flow diagram*

The HACCP team should confirm the processing operation against the flow diagram during all stages and hours of operation and amend the flow diagram where appropriate.

6. *List all potential hazards associated with each step, conduct a hazard analysis, and consider any measures to control identified hazards*

The HACCP team should list all possible hazards that can occur at each step. The HACCP team should then conduct a hazard analysis to identify for the HACCP plan which hazards should be considered a priority (i.e., the hazards that are of such a nature that their elimination or reduction to acceptable levels is essential to the production of safe food).

In conducting the hazard analysis, wherever possible the following should be included:

- the likely occurrence of hazards and severity of their adverse health effects
- the qualitative and/or quantitative evaluation of the presence of hazards
- survival or multiplication of microorganisms of concern
- production or persistence in foods of toxins, chemicals, or physical agents
- conditions that lead to the above

The HACCP team must then consider what control measures, if any, exist that can be applied to each hazard. More than one control measure might be necessary to control a specific hazard(s), and more than one hazard might be controlled by a specified control measure.

7. *Determine critical control points*

The determination of a CCP in the HACCP system can be facilitated by the application of a decision tree. Decision trees can be used to indicate a logic reasoning approach and should be flexible to be widely applicable (i.e., used to determine CCPs in the various steps of operation, such as production, slaughter, processing, storage, distribution, etc.). Training in the application of the decision tree is recommended.

If a hazard has been identified at a step where control is necessary for safety, and no control measure exists at that step or any other, then the product or process should be modified at

FIGURE 12.2   Example of Decision Tree to Identify CCPs

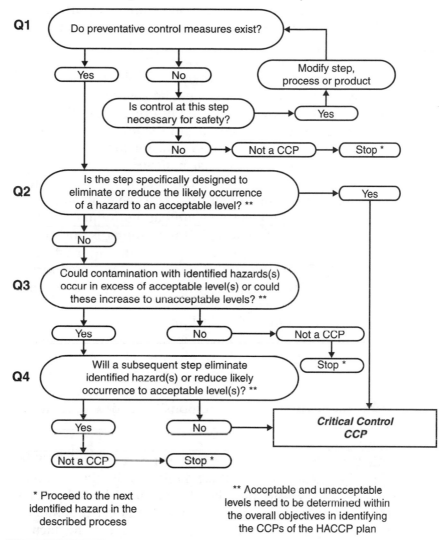

* Proceed to the next
identified hazard in the
described process

** Acceptable and unacceptable
levels need to be determined within
the overall objectives in identifying
the CCPs of the HACCP plan

Source: World Health Organization. Retrieved December 27, 2007, from http://www.who.int/
foodsafety/fs_management/en/intro_haccp_figures.pdf.

that step, or at any earlier or later stage, to include a control
measure.

8. *Establish critical limits for each CCP*
Critical limits must be specified and validated if possible for
each CCP. In some cases more than one critical limit will be

elaborated at a particular step. Criteria often used include measurements of temperature, time, moisture level, pH, Aw, available chlorine, and sensory parameters such as visual appearance and texture.

9. *Establish a monitoring system for each CCP*
Monitoring, the scheduled measurement or observation of a CCP relative to its critical limits, must be able to detect loss of control at the CCP as well as provide information in time to make adjustments to ensure control of the process to prevent violating the critical limits. Process adjustments should be made when monitoring results that indicate a trend toward loss of control at a CCP and should be taken before a deviation occurs. Data derived from monitoring must be evaluated by a designated person with knowledge and authority to carry out corrective actions when indicated. If monitoring is not continuous, then the amount or frequency of monitoring must be sufficient to guarantee the CCP is in control. Most monitoring procedures for CCPs will need to be done rapidly because they relate to online processes, and there will not be time for lengthy analytical testing. Physical and chemical measurements are often preferred to microbiological testing because they can be done rapidly and can often indicate the microbiological control of the product. All records and documents associated with monitoring CCPs must be signed by the person(s) doing the monitoring and by a responsible reviewing official(s) of the company.

10. *Establish corrective actions*
Specific corrective actions must be developed for each CCP in the HACCP system to deal with deviations when they occur. The actions must ensure that the CCP has been brought under control, including proper disposition of the affected product. Deviation and product disposition procedures must be documented in the HACCP record keeping.

11. *Establish verification procedures*
Verification and auditing methods, procedures, and tests, including random sampling and analysis, can be used to determine if the HACCP system is working correctly. The frequency of verification should be sufficient to confirm that the HACCP system is working effectively. Examples of verification activities include:

- review of the HACCP system and its records
- review of deviations and product dispositions
- confirmation that CCPs are kept under control

Where possible, validation activities should include actions to confirm the efficacy of all elements of the HACCP plan.

12. *Establish documentation and record keeping*
Efficient and accurate record keeping is essential to the application of an HACCP system. Documentation and record keeping should be appropriate to the nature and size of the operation.
Documentation examples are:

- hazard analysis
- CCP determination
- critical limit determination

Record examples are:

- CCP monitoring activities
- deviations and associated corrective actions
- modifications to the HACCP system

Learning Point: Training of personnel in industry, government, and academia in HACCP principles and applications and increasing awareness of consumers are essential elements for the effective implementation of HACCP. Working instructions and procedures should be developed that define the tasks of the operating personnel to be stationed at each CCP. Opportunities should also be provided for the joint training of industry and control authorities to encourage and maintain a continuous dialog and create a climate of understanding in the practical application of HACCP.

HACCP and Regulatory Oversight

In addition to the enhancement of food safety, HACCP can provide other significant benefits. For example, the application of HACCP systems can aid inspection and regulatory agencies, such as the FDA and the USDA, and promote international trade by increasing confidence in food safety.

The USDA and HACCP

In 1996, the USDA's FSIS published the Pathogen Reduction: Hazard Analysis and Critical Control Point (HACCP) Systems (PR/HACCP) final rule (USDA, 1997). The new final rule on Pathogen Reduction and HACCP Systems consists of 183 pages of regulations. The rule mandates new measures in slaughter and processing plants to target and reduce the presence of pathogenic organisms in meat and poultry products. The seven HACCP principles recommended by the NACMCF in 1992 provided the framework for the PR/HACCP final rule. The new rule was the result of the necessity to modernize the USDA inspection system from a visual one, based only on what FSIS inspectors could see (e.g., evidence of animal diseases, defects, and visible contamination on meat) to a scientific system, based on the prevention of hazards and regular microbial testing. This need became urgent when, in January 1993, a widely publicized outbreak of the bacteria *E. coli* O157:H7 struck more than 500 people and resulted in four deaths (Davis, et al., 1993). This potentially deadly strain of bacteria was traced to hamburger meat that had been distributed throughout the western states.. The importance of the final rule was the fact that it placed the responsibility for such foodborne disease outbreaks (FBDOs) appropriately with industry.

Implementation of the final rule began in 1997 and required that all inspected facilities have in place written Sanitation Standard Operating Procedures (SSOPs). Phase one of the HACCP implementation began in January 1998 in all large plants that slaughter and/or process meat or poultry. On January 26, 1998, these plants were required to have both written HACCP plans and operating HACCP systems. Establishments' HACCP plans must meet five regulatory features including: (1) monitoring; (2) verification; (3) record keeping; (4) corrective actions; and (5) reassessment. In addition to requiring the development of HACCP plans, the final rule included a number of requirements for pathogen reduction in meat and poultry products. For example, all establishments that slaughter animals or ship raw ground product were required to meet pathogen reduction performance standards for *Salmonella*. The purpose of the *Salmonella* performance standards was to provide both incentives for producers of raw meat and poultry products to reduce the prevalence of *Salmonella* on their products and to provide an objective basis for judging the effectiveness of establishments' HACCP plans by both FSIS and establishments. All slaughter establishments were also required to implement generic *Escherichia coli* testing programs. This microbial testing by slaughter establishments can be used to verify the adequacy of the establishment's process controls for the prevention and removal of fecal contamination and associated bacteria. In addition, CCPs to eliminate contamination with visible fecal material were to be included as essential components of all slaughter establishments' HACCP plans. To implement an HACCP plan for each of their processes, the potential hazards associated with incoming animals must be considered. The need for background information on incoming animals will have an effect on the entire chain of food animal production. Information about the source of the animal; the selection, timing, and use of animal drugs; and documentation of a valid veterinary–client–patient relationship for prescription and extra-label drug use will help with the evaluation of risks and help to ensure the safety of product leaving the plant. These three components—valid HACCP systems assuring compliance with the food safety standards, such as the zero fecal contamination; compliance with *Salmonella* performance standards by establishments that slaughter or ship raw ground products; and generic *E. coli* testing programs conducted by slaughter establishments—were designed to provide an integrated approach to process control and pathogen reduction. The next three phases of the HACCP implementation plan were scheduled according to plant size. During the next two consecutive years, small plants and very small plants, respectively, were bound to the same requirements.

Under the new HACCP guidelines, the roles and responsibilities of both industry and government were explicitly clarified. According to these guidelines, FSIS's main role is to set appropriate food safety standards and maintain vigorous inspection oversight and verification to help ensure that those standards were being met. Establishments must have preventive HACCP systems in place to ensure the production of safe and unadulterated food. They are required to monitor and verify the performance of the controls in their HACCP plans and to maintain records of this monitoring and verification. FSIS inspects these systems, and the products from official establishments are labeled with the mark of inspection. This mark indicates that they have been inspected and are eligible for sale and transportation in commerce. When establishments fail to develop or carry out effective HACCP systems, FSIS takes action to control products by withholding or suspending inspection. Withholding the mark of inspection effectively shuts down affected operations because it is illegal to sell products in interstate commerce that do not bear the USDA mark of inspection. As a result of this clarification of responsibility, FSIS inspection personnel perform inspection procedures designed to verify an HACCP plan's basic compliance with regulatory requirements, the effectiveness of an establishment's HACCP plan(s), and whether the establishment meets pathogen reduction standards. Verification of an establishment's HACCP plan is made through observation and review of the establishment's records. If regulatory requirements are not met or an establishment fails to maintain its control systems properly, the noncompliance is documented and, as needed, appropriate regulatory action is taken. Additionally, inspection personnel conduct *Salmonella* sampling in establishments that slaughter animals or ship raw ground products.

With the implementation of the PR/HACCP final rule in January 1997, food safety moved away from a command-and-control philosophy to one that emphasized separation of government and industry roles and performance standards for industry. These changes have had an affect on inspection policies and practices among all government employees. To overcome the new challenges to the inspection workforce, FSIS provided an Introductory HACCP Technical Training Program for all FSIS employees. In addition to providing technical training for its personnel, FSIS established the Technical Service Center (TSC). TSC, which is accessible by telephone, fax, or e-mail, was set up as a central information source for employees and industry to answer technical questions regarding any aspect of inspection. The purpose of the TSC was to address the need for accurate and consistent distribution of information, correlate the execution of inspection procedures and requirements, and lead the implementation of new and modified inspection programs and procedures. An HACCP Hotline was also established to answer employees' and industry's questions specifically related to Phase One implementation of the PR/HACCP final rule. These resources were set up to address the need for accurate and consistent distribution of information, correlate the execution of inspection procedures and requirements, and lead the implementation of new and modified inspection programs and procedures.

The FDA and HACCP

New challenges to the US food supply have prompted the FDA to consider adopting an HACCP-based food safety system on a wider basis (FDA, 2001b). One of the most important challenges is the increasing number of new food pathogens. For example, between 1973 and 1988, bacteria not previously recognized as important causes of foodborne illness, such as *E. coli* O157:H7 and *Salmonella enteritidis*, became more widespread. There are also increasing public health concerns about chemical contamination of food, such as the effects of lead in food on the nervous system. Another important factor is the size of the food industry and the diversity of products and processes. At the same time, the FDA and state and local agencies have the same limited level of resources to ensure food safety. The need for HACCP in the United States is further fueled by the growing trend in international trade for worldwide equivalence of food products and the Codex Alimentarius Commission's adoption of HACCP as the international standard for food safety. These challenges have made the traditional methods of regulation obsolete. Industry and regulators have traditionally depended on spot checks of manufacturing conditions and random sampling of final products to ensure food safety; however, these methods tend to be reactive and have proven to be ineffective. HACCP is proactive, and many of its principles are already in place in the FDA-regulated low-acid canned food industry. The FDA also established HACCP for the seafood industry in 1995 and for the juice industry in 2001. Furthermore, the FDA is now considering the development of regulations that would establish HACCP as the food safety standard throughout other areas of the food industry, including both domestic and imported food products.

Juice HACCP

The presence of some of the pathogens (i.e., *E. coli* O157:H7 and *Cryptosporidium*) that have been responsible for recent outbreaks of foodborne illness associated with untreated juice products is a relatively new phenomenon (Lewis, 1999). Therefore, consumers do not associate such pathogens, and the risk that they present, with the consumption of untreated juice. In contrast, consumers have some awareness that meat and poultry products have the potential to contain harmful microorganisms. Also, these foods ordinarily are cooked prior to consumption. Moreover, meat and poultry products that are regulated by the USDA's FSIS are subject to that agency's HACCP regulations.

A 1997 study by the FDA's Center for Food Safety and Applied Nutrition (CFSAN) found that while contamination of juice products most likely occurs during the growing and harvesting of the raw product, it can occur at any point between the orchard and the table. Therefore, the FDA's proposed regulation will require juice processors to implement an HACCP plan that addresses all points of production. In the 1997 study, recombinant *E. coli* O157:H7 growth in apple juice and orange juice indicated that these juices do provide an environment for growth of this organism. In the study, there was only a small decline in numbers of *E. coli* O157:H7 inoculated into orange juice over a 24-day period at refrigeration temperatures. The fact that *E. coli* O157:H7 can survive in citrus juice and the fact that human illnesses from other pathogens have been traced epidemiologically to citrus juice demonstrates that, if contaminated, these juices have potential to cause human illness. The knowledge that *E. coli* and other pathogens have been found in juice and have caused illness indicates that a processor must take steps (i.e., pathogen reduction steps to achieve the performance standard) to ensure that the juice is safe, regardless of its source. These steps must include prevention of contamination, destruction of any pathogens of concern that might be present, or both. If future research determines new sources of *E. coli* O157:H7 or other pathogens in juice products, processors could then develop appropriate measures to prevent contamination from these sources and apply measures that are determined to be effective toward the pathogen reduction performance standard.

Based on information collected in the wake of these outbreaks, the FDA determined that the use of good manufacturing practices (GMP) and FDA inspections were not enough to adequately address the safety of fresh juices. Therefore, in 1997, the FDA published a notice of intent that announced a comprehensive program to address the incidence of foodborne illness related to consumption of fresh juice and ultimately to address the safety of all juice products. According to the notice of intent, the FDA would initiate a rulemaking on a mandatory HACCP program for some or all juice products; propose that the labels of juice products that are not specifically processed to prevent, reduce, or eliminate pathogens bear a warning statement informing consumers of the risk of illness associated with consumption of the product; and initiate several educational programs to minimize the hazards associated with consumption of fresh juices.

As a result of the recent outbreaks associated with juices, the FDA announced a final rule designed to improve the safety of fruit and vegetable juices. The rule comes in the wake of a rise in the number of foodborne illness outbreaks and consumer illnesses associated with juice products, including a 1999 *E. coli* O157:H7 outbreak associated with apple juice products and two citrus juice outbreaks associated with *Salmonella* spp. in 1999 and 2000. Some of the illnesses associated with these outbreaks have been very severe (e.g., cases of long-term reactive arthritis and severe chronic illness); in one case, consumption of contaminated juice resulted in death. As is the case with most food-associated disease, it is assumed that these outbreaks represent a fraction of the outbreaks and sporadic cases that actually occur. The FDA estimates that there are between 16,000 to 48,000 cases of juice-related illnesses each year, and application of the new rule is expected to reduce these numbers by at least 6000.

Prior to implementation of HACCP regulations by the FDA for juices, the Fresh Produce Subcommittee (FPS) of the National Advisory Committee on Microbiological Criteria for Foods (NACMCF) met in a drafting session in 1996 to consider the safety of all juices (FDA, 1997). The FPS risk conclusions were based on documented outbreaks of illness associated with consumption of contaminated juices. According to the FPS, many aspects affect pathogen control, including agricultural practices, product handling, equipment used, growing location (e.g., below ground, on ground, from trees), pH, acidulants, methods of processing, degree of animal contact, refrigeration, packaging, and the distribution system (FDA, 1997). On the basis of all the testimony presented at this meeting, the FSP members agreed that there was a need to understand the differences among all juice and juice products (e.g., citrus versus others). They also identified the means to clearly differentiate between unpasteurized and pasteurized products as a significant problem. According to the committee, the terms used to identify juice products do not always have universal meanings (e.g., the term "cider" is perceived to be an unpasteurized product whereas the term "juice" is often perceived to be pasteurized). Furthermore, they determined that the history of public health problems associated with fresh juices indicated a need for active safety interventions and recommended mandatory HACCP for all juice products.

The FDA published its final rule for implementation of HACCP in the juice industry in 2001. The juice HACCP regulations apply to juice products in both interstate and intrastate commerce (FDA, 2001a). Juice processors, under the new guidelines, will be required to evaluate their manufacturing process to determine whether there are any microbiological, chemical, or physical hazards that could contaminate their products. If a potential hazard is identified, processors will be required to implement control measures to prevent, reduce, or eliminate the hazard. Processors are also required to use processes that achieve a 5-log, or 100,000-fold, reduction in the numbers of the most resistant pathogens in their finished products compared to levels that might be present in untreated juice. Juice processors can use microbial reduction methods other than pasteurization, such as UV irradiation technology and other approved alternative technologies, or a combination of techniques. Citrus juice processors can opt to apply the 5-log pathogen reduction rule on the surface of the fruit in combination with microbial testing to assure that this process is effective. Processors that make shelf-stable juices or concentrates that use a single thermal processing step are exempt from the microbial hazard requirements of the HACCP regulation. Retail establishments where packaged juice is made and only sold directly to consumers (e.g., juice bars) are not required to comply with this regulation.

Deadlines were established by the FDA for implementation of the new rule. Large companies had one year after the publication of the regulation to implement HACCP programs. Small companies had two years after the publication, and very small companies had three years after publication. All companies were required to post warning label statements on their products until they implemented the HACCP programs. In the interim, the FDA continued to inspect juice processing facilities to assure that they were producing safe juice and juice products.

Seafood HACCP

Several outbreaks have been associated with contaminated seafood (Kurtzweil, 1997). For example, in 1997, 26 employees of a Washington, DC bank became ill as a result of consuming scombroid-contaminated blue marlin in their workplace cafeteria. Seafood can be exposed to a range of hazards, many of which are natural to seafood's environment, and include bacteria, viruses, parasites, natural toxins, and chemical contaminants.

The FDA's seafood HACCP program applies to both imported and domestically produced seafood (FDA, 2005). The majority of all seafood consumed in the United States is imported. About 160 countries import seafood into the United States, only some of which have advanced regulatory systems for seafood. The traditional strategy has been to review entries of import products into the United States and to select products for physical examination at ports of entry. The examinations are primarily directed toward determining whether the product contains substances that would cause it to be adulterated under US law. This examination would not necessarily reveal whether the products were produced under HACCP-type preventive controls in the country of origin. Consequently, the FDA determined that new strategies to augment port of entry examinations were necessary. The first strategy was a requirement in the Seafood HACCP Regulation that US importers take "affirmative steps" to help ensure that imported seafood products have been processed in accordance with the US HACCP requirements. Affirmative steps can be basic, threshold indicators of performance, such as obtaining copies of foreign processors' HACCP plans and records. The second strategy in the regulations required a significant increase in foreign regulatory inspections by FDA inspectors. Many of these inspections have been directed toward developing countries that are major exporters of seafood, such as Vietnam. These countries were chosen by the FDA because they are less likely to provide advanced, HACCP-based regulatory feedback to their own processors than highly developed countries. Countries with advanced regulatory systems for seafood are generally implementing and enforcing HACCP-based systems for their products.

In 2002 and 2003, the FDA sent inspection teams to 11 and 7 countries, respectively, that are major exporters of seafood into the United States. The objective was to engage in direct, in-plant compliance inspections of foreign processors and to develop contacts and relationships with the competent inspection authorities and industries in these countries. The FDA also wanted to provide training and educational opportunities to both industry and government. While on these trips, the FDA discovered several important distinctions between US and foreign inspections that make comparisons difficult: (1) foreign inspections are performed on different firms and in different countries from year to year, while domestic inspections are performed on the same firms; (2) foreign inspections focus on products with an elevated food safety risk, while domestic inspections cover products across the risk spectrum; (3) foreign inspections tend to focus on firms with regulatory problems, while such firms make up only a relatively small portion of those covered domestically; and (4) foreign inspections are announced months in advance, whereas domestic inspections are unannounced.

The FDA established HACCP for the seafood industry in a final rule on December 18, 1995. The safety features of the FDA's HACCP regulations were incorporated into the National Seafood Inspection Program of the Department of Commerce's National Oceanic and Atmospheric Administration (NOAA). For a fee, the NOAA inspects seafood processors and others, checking vessels and plants for sanitation and examining product quality. The agency certifies seafood plants that meet federal standards and rates products with grades based on their quality. Seafood processors in good standing with the program are free to use official marks on their products to indicate that the seafood has been federally inspected. The FDA has also included additional protections to promote seafood safety in other ways, including the following:

- Setting standards for seafood contaminants, such as legally binding safety limits for polychlorinated biphenyls and guidelines for safety limits for six pesticides, mercury, paralytic shellfish poison, and histamine (the chemical responsible for scombroid poisoning).
- Administration of the National Shellfish Sanitation Program, which involves 23 shellfish-producing states, plus a few non-shellfish-producing states, and nine countries. This program exercises control over all sanitation related to the growing, harvesting, shucking, packing, and interstate transportation of oysters, clams, and other molluscan shellfish.
- Lending expertise to the Interstate Shellfish Sanitation Conference (an organization of federal and state agencies and members of the shellfish industry) to aid in the development of uniform guidelines and procedures for state agencies to monitor shellfish safety.

- Entering into cooperative programs with states to provide training to state and local health officials who inspect fishing areas, seafood processing plants and warehouses, and restaurants and other retail places.
- Working with NOAA to close federal waters to fishing whenever oil spills, toxic blooms, or other phenomena threaten seafood safety.
- Sampling and analyzing fish and fishery products for toxins, chemicals, and other hazards in agency laboratories.

International HACCP Alliance

The International HACCP Alliance, formerly known as the International Meat and Poultry HACCP Alliance, was established in 1994 to assist the meat and poultry industry in preparing for mandatory HACCP (International HACCP Alliance, 2007). Since March 1994, the HACCP Alliance has focused on standardizing HACCP training efforts, developing a uniform position for the implementation of HACCP, and collaborative efforts with the USDA's Food Safety and Inspection Service (FSIS) and other regulatory agencies. As a result of their efforts, five standardized curricula have been developed, more than 25 training programs have been accredited, and more than 100 individuals have been approved as lead instructors. As of this writing, the HACCP Alliance membership includes members from numerous other countries, including the United States, Canada, Australia, Argentina, Mexico, etc., that represent industry associations, professional associations, educational foundations, universities, third party/private companies, and government cooperators.

The HACCP Alliance recognizes the importance of food safety as a critical component of both public health and economic growth. Therefore, their goal is to facilitate the uniform development and implementation of HACCP programs from farm to table. To accomplish this goal, the HACCP Alliance provides a forum where issues are deliberated and resolved uniformly to assure that food safety plans are effective and sufficient throughout the entire commercial food chain system.

The goals of the International HACCP Alliance are as follows:

- to be recognized as the worldwide HACCP authority
- to provide standardized curricula and accreditation for HACCP/food safety courses

- to facilitate the standardization of support systems for HACCP
- to foster understanding and cooperation among industry, academia, consumers, and government regarding HACCP and food safety

There is a wide variety of seafood in US seafood markets and grocery stores (e.g., crabs and clams, bass, red snapper, catfish, octopus and squid, mackerel and salmon, to name a few). This variety, from a food safety perspective, allows for a wide variety of contaminants. According to the FDA, the establishment of HACCP in the seafood industry, along with ongoing research and other federal and state activities as well as careful handling by consumers, can help ensure that the seafood not only tastes good and is healthy but is safe as well.

The Food and Agriculture Organization of the United Nations (FAO) and the World Health Organization (WHO)

The Codex Alimentarius, Latin for "food code," is a collection of internationally recognized standards, codes of practices, guidelines, and other recommendations relating to foods, food production, and food safety under the aegis of consumer protection (Food and Agriculture Organization of the United Nations and the World Health Organization, 1999; Food and Agriculture Organization of the United Nations and the World Health Organization, 2006). These texts are developed and maintained by the Codex Alimentarius Commission, a body that was established by the FAO and the WHO in 1963. The commission's main objective is to protect the health of consumers and ensure fair practices in the international food trade.

The Codex Alimentarius officially covers all foods that are marketed directly to consumers, whether processed, semiprocessed, or raw. In addition to the standards for specific foods, the Codex Alimentarius contains general guidelines for food labeling, food hygiene, food additives and pesticide residues, and procedures for assessing the safety of foods derived from modern biotechnology. It also contains guidelines for the management of governmental import and export inspections and certification systems for foods. These guidelines are published on the Codex Alimentarius Web site in various languages, including Arabic, Chinese, English, French, and Spanish.

In the Codex General Principles of Food Hygiene, the Codex Alimentarius Commission recommends an HACCP-based approach as a means of enhancing food safety. The committee also provides guidelines for the implementation of HACCP principles. At the 35th Session of the Codex Committee on Food Hygiene in 2003, it was agreed that the Food and Agriculture Organization (FAO) of the United Nations and the World Health Organization (WHO) would develop HACCP guidelines for small and/or less developed businesses (SLDBs). In 2004, FAO/WHO convened an electronic discussion group of experts with experience in the area of food safety and/or food production. The information gathered from this meeting was used to prepare the first draft of the HACCP guidelines. The FAO and WHO support the continual development of national policies to improve food safety and quality with the overall objective of protecting consumers' health and furthering economic development.

Chapter Summary

As mentioned before, the HACCP system is a preventive approach to food safety. It is based on the application of scientific principles to food processing and production and has been in use by the food industry since the 1970s. The primary advantage of the HACCP system includes the following:

- it focuses on identifying and preventing hazards from contaminating foods
- it is based on sound science
- it permits more efficient and effective government oversight, primarily because the record keeping allows investigators to see how well a firm complies with food safety laws over a period rather than how well it is doing on any given day
- it places the responsibility for ensuring food safety appropriately on the food manufacturer or distributor
- it helps food companies compete more effectively in the world market
- it reduces barriers to international trade

HACCP has been implemented by the USDA in all plants that slaughter and/or process meat or poultry. HACCP has been implemented by the FDA in both the juice industry and the seafood industry. The Codex Alimentarius Commission, a body that was established by the FAO and the WHO in 1963, recommends an HACCP-based approach as a means of enhancing food safety for all its affiliated countries.

Issues to Debate

1. Do you think that the HACCP system will prove to be more effective than traditional food safety systems? Explain why or why not.
2. How and why is scientific knowledge important in the development of HACCP plans?
3. Critical control points are considered to be one of the most important aspects of HACCP systems. Why is this, and what are some of the major areas in which these points can occur?
4. Since HACCP was developed in 1959, why do you think it took so long for government agencies and industry to consider its use?
5. Since HACCP has been in use in several areas of food production, such as the meat and poultry industries, juice industry, and seafood industry, do you think that it has led to a reduction in foodborne illnesses? Explain why or why not.

References

Davis, M., Osaki, C., Gordon, D., Hinds, M. W., Mottram, K., Winegar, C., et al. (1993). Update: Multistate outbreak of *Escherichia coli* O157:H7 infections from hamburgers–Western United States, 1992–1993. *Morbidity and Mortality Weekly Report, 42,* 258–263.

Food and Agriculture Organization of the United Nations and the World Health Organization. (1998). *Guidance on regulatory assessment of HACCP: Report of a joint FAO/WHO consultation on the role of government agencies in assessing HACCP.* Retrieved October 24, 2007, from http://www.who.int

Food and Agriculture Organization of the United Nations and the World Health Organization. (1999). *Codex Alimentarius: Food hygiene basic texts* (2nd ed.). Retrieved October 20, 2007, from http://www.fao.org

Food and Agriculture Organization of the United Nations and the World Health Organization. (2006). *Understanding the Codex Alimentarius* (3rd ed.). Retrieved October 30, 2007, from http://www.fao.org

Food and Drug Administration. (1997). *Recommendations on fresh juice.* Retrieved October 20, 2007, from http://www.cfsan.fda.gov

Food and Drug Administration. (2001a). *FDA publishes final rule to increase safety of fruit and vegetable juices.* Retrieved October 12, 2007, from http://www.cfsan.fda.gov

Food and Drug Administration. (2001b). *HACCP: A state-of-the-art approach to food safety.* Retrieved October 15, 2007, from http://www.cfsan.fda.gov

Food and Drug Administration. (2005). *FDA's evaluation of the seafood HACCP programs for fiscal years 2002/2003.* Retrieved October 15, 2007, from http://www.cfsan.fda.gov

International HACCP Alliance. (2007). *International HACCP alliance.* Retrieved October 15, 2007, from http://www.haccpalliance.org

Kurtzweil, P. (1997). *Critical steps toward safer seafood.* Retrieved October 15, 2007, from http://www.cfsan.fda.gov

Lewis, C. (1999). *Critical controls for juice safety.* Retrieved October 12, 2007, from http://www.cfsan.fda.gov

US Department of Agriculture. (1997). *HACCP implementation (June 1997).* Retrieved October 20, 2007, from http://fsis.usda.gov

US Department of Agriculture. (2007). *National Advisory Committee on Microbiological Criteria for Foods.* Retrieved October 20, 2007, from http://www.fsis.usda.gov

CHAPTER 13

US FOOD SAFETY AND BIOTERRORISM

Tamara M. Crutchley Bushell, PhD

Chapter Objectives

After reading the chapter and reflecting on the contents, you should be able to:

1. Describe the collaborative efforts needed to improve food safety.
2. Explain how enactment of the bills passed after 9/11 might improve food safety.
3. Discuss what the different government agencies are doing to improve food safety.
4. Discuss what the different academic institutions are doing to improve food safety.
5. Discuss what industry is doing to improve food safety.

Key Terms

agriculture: The process of producing food, feed, fiber, fuel, and other goods by the systematic raising of plants and animals.

agroterrorism: The malicious use of plant or animal pathogens to cause devastating disease in agriculture.

collaboration: The process by which people and organizations work together to accomplish a common mission.

food chain: The pathway along which food is transferred from food producers to food consumers.

food research: The careful, systematic study, investigation, and compilation of information about foods and their components.

food safety: A scientific discipline that describes the handling, preparation, and storage of food in ways that prevent foodborne illness.

food technology: The application of food science to the selection, preservation, processing, packaging, distribution, and use of safe, nutritious, and wholesome food.

preparedness: The activities and measures taken in advance to ensure effective response to the impact of hazards.

presidential directive: A directive issued by the president of the United States, usually addressed to all heads of departments and agencies.

prevention: The act of preventing or impeding.

risk reduction: Consists of the selective application of appropriate techniques and management principles to reduce either the likelihood of occurrence or its impact, or both.

Introduction

According to public health and food safety experts, each year tens of millions of illnesses in the United States can be traced to foodborne pathogens. The symptoms of the illnesses range from mild gastroenteritis to life-threatening neurologic, hepatic, and renal syndromes. The FDA estimates that 2% to 3% of the illnesses traced to foodborne pathogens result in secondary long-term illnesses. For example, certain strains of *Escherichia coli* can cause kidney failure in young children and infants; *Salmonella* can lead to reactive arthritis and serious infections; *Listeria* can cause meningitis and stillbirths; and *Campylobacter* can be a precipitating factor for Guillain-Barre syndrome. These types of food safety issues will continue to generate the need for change, both to respond to public concerns and to provide policy makers with scientific data as a basis for sound, reasoned judgments. As new and creative foods become more common, continuing efforts will need a strong foundation to assess the complexity of interactions of food components as they relate to food safety. To this end, industry, the scientific community, and government need to realize that further improvements can be made through collaborative efforts based on the following:

- the use of science-based pathogen intervention strategies to enhance sanitary processes that include effective and microbiological verifiable HACCP
- the principles of prevention and risk reduction from the farm to fork that include effective monitoring and intervention strategies

- the understanding by each segment of the food chain of the food safety risks affected by production and the steps needed to ensure safety

Every segment of industry needs to unite behind effective programs aimed immediately at solving the problem of current food safety issues. Industry must also strive to align the programs and policies of the government to support and enhance these efforts. This effort requires that everyone involved rethink their current approaches to food safety and adopt new strategies and collaborative efforts designed to support a comprehensive system spanning the entire food continuum.

What Government Agencies Are Doing to Improve Food Safety

Several bills have been enacted that address some aspect of food safety. For example, the Public Health Security and Bioterrorism Preparedness and Response Act (Bioterrorism Act) of 2002 was signed into law by President Bush on June 12, 2002 (Food and Drug Administration, 2002). The Bioterrorism Act directs the secretary of the US Department of Health and Human Services (HHS) to develop and implement a coordinated strategy, building upon core public health capabilities established under provisions of the act, for carrying out health-related activities to prepare for and respond effectively to bioterrorism and other public health emergencies. Under these new guidelines, the secretary of HHS is supplied with new authorities to protect the nation's food supply against the threat of intentional contamination as well as other food-related emergencies. For example, Title III of the Bioterrorism Act deals specifically with agricultural security by increasing inspection capacity at points of origin, improving surveillance at ports of entry, and enhancing methods of protecting against bioterrorism. As part of this provision, the Secretary is authorized to:

1. Set forth reporting requirements and authorize appropriations (Section 302).
2. Permit an officer or qualified employee of the US Food and Drug Administration (FDA) to order the temporary detention of any article of food if the officer or qualified employee finds,

during an inspection, examination, or investigation, credible evidence or information indicating that such article presents a threat of serious adverse health consequences or death to humans or animals (Section 303).

3. Provide for the debarment of importers for repeated or serious food import violations (Section 304).
4. Require that any facility (domestic and foreign) engaged in manufacturing, processing, packing, or holding food for consumption in the United States be registered with the secretary (Section 305).
5. Require that access be permitted to all records needed to assist the secretary in determining whether food is adulterated and presents a threat of serious adverse health consequences or death to humans or animals (Section 306).
6. Require that all food importers give the secretary specified prior notice (including specified information about the source of food) of the importation of any food for the purpose of enabling the food to be inspected (Section 307).
7. Require that the owner or consignee of food refused admission into the United States, but not ordered to be destroyed, affix to the container of the food a label that clearly and conspicuously bears the statement: United States: Refused Entry (Section 308).
8. Prohibit an importer from port shopping with respect to food that has previously been denied entry (Section 309).
9. Provide notice regarding threats associated with a shipment of imported food to the appropriate states (Section 310).
10. Allocate funds to states, territories, and Indian tribes to assist with the costs of enhancing food safety efforts as well as costs associated with examinations, inspections, and investigations where a credible threat of adulterated food is present (Sections 311 and 312).
11. Coordinate zoonotic disease surveillance (Section 313).
12. Commission officers and qualified employees of other federal departments or federal agencies to conduct examinations and inspections for the secretary under the Federal Food, Drug, and Cosmetic Act. Subtitle B of Title II directs the secretary of agriculture to establish and maintain a list of each biological agent and each toxin that the secretary determines has the potential

to pose a severe threat to animal or plant health or to animal or plant products.

Subtitle D of Title II amends the federal criminal code provisions concerning the possession of listed biological agents and toxins to provide that whoever transfers a select agent to a person who the transferor knows or has reasonable cause to believe is not registered as required shall be fined, imprisoned for not more than 5 years, or both; if a person knowingly possesses a biological agent or toxin where such agent or toxin is a select agent for which such person has not obtained a required registration shall be fined, imprisoned for not more than 5 years, or both.

The Homeland Security Act of 2002 was enacted as a direct result of the 9/11 terrorist attacks (Homeland Security Act, 2006). The primary purpose of the Homeland Security Act was to create the Department of Homeland Security (DHS). The DHS was established under Section 101 of the guidelines as an executive department of the United States, headed by a Secretary of Homeland Security appointed by the president, to:

1. Prevent terrorist attacks within the United States.
2. Reduce the vulnerability of the United States to terrorism.
3. Minimize the damage, and assist in the recovery, from terrorist attacks within the United States.
4. Carry out all functions of entities transferred to the DHS.
5. Ensure that the functions of the agencies and subdivisions within the DHS that are not related directly to securing the homeland are not diminished or neglected except by a specific Act of Congress.
6. Ensure that the overall economic security of the United States is not diminished by efforts, activities, and programs aimed at securing the homeland.
7. Monitor connections between illegal drug trafficking and terrorism, coordinate efforts to sever such connections, and otherwise contribute to efforts to interdict illegal drug trafficking.

Under Section 202 of the guidelines, all federal agencies must promptly supply the secretary of the DHS with:

1. all reports, assessments, and analytical information related to threats of terrorism and to other responsibilities assigned to the secretary

2. all information concerning the vulnerability of the US infrastructure or other US vulnerabilities to terrorism, whether or not it has been analyzed
3. all other information related to significant and credible threats of terrorism, whether or not it has been analyzed
4. such other information or material as the president may direct

As part of the largest governmental reorganization in 50 years, the DHS assumed a number of government functions previously conducted by other departments, such as agricultural border inspection, functions under the US Customs Service, and functions under the Transportation Security Administration. Possession of the Plum Island Animal Disease Center in New York was also transferred to the DHS. As a result of the reorganization, the DHS is now the third largest cabinet department in the US federal government, after the Department of Defense and the Department of Veterans Affairs.

Two presidential directives with direct ties to food safety were passed as a result of enactment of the Homeland Security Act of 2002. Homeland Security Presidential Directive-9 was signed by President Bush in 2004 to establish a national policy to defend the agriculture and food system against terrorist attacks, major disasters, and other emergencies by requiring actions in the following areas:

1. awareness and warning
2. vulnerability assessments
3. mitigation strategies
4. response planning and recovery
5. outreach and professional development
6. research and development (Federation of American Scientists, 2004; Nolen, 2004)

Homeland Security Presidential Directive-7 made the DHS responsible for coordinating the overall national effort to enhance the protection of the critical infrastructure and key resources of the United States (White House, 2003). An important issue in Homeland Security Presidential Directive-9 is the focus on veterinary medicine as a critical component of food security. For example, the policy calls for the creation of a national stockpile of animal drugs and vaccines to better respond to serious animal diseases; grants to veterinary colleges for expanding training in exotic animal diseases, epidemiology, and public health; and inclusion of veterinary diagnostic laboratories in national networks of federal and state laboratories. Ultimately, the goal of implementing this directive is the development of a robust, comprehensive, and fully coordinated surveillance and monitoring system for public and animal health. The policy also directs the Departments of Agriculture, Health and Human Services, and Homeland Security to establish internships, fellowships, and other postgraduate opportunities for professional development and specialized training in agriculture and food protection that provide for homeland security professional workforce needs. If implemented in its entirety, this document will have a long-standing and positive influence on animal health and animal agriculture.

As a result of the previously mentioned legislation, federal and state agencies have implemented initiatives to address agricultural and food defense issues. Since its inception, the DHS has focused its efforts on a six-point agenda (Food and Drug Administration, 2004; US Department of Homeland Security, 2006):

1. to increase overall preparedness
2. to create better transportation security systems
3. to strengthen border security
4. to enhance information sharing
5. to improve financial management
6. to realign the DHS organization to maximize mission performance

The National Preparedness System was developed within the DHS as part of this agenda (Dyckman, 2003). This system was designed to provide a comprehensive assessment of national preparedness and has six basic components:

1. The National Preparedness Goal, which sets a general goal for national preparedness, identifies the means of measuring such preparedness and establishes national preparedness priorities.
2. Fifteen planning scenarios set forth as examples of catastrophic situations to which nonfederal agencies are expected to be able to respond.
3. The Universal Task List, which identifies specific tasks that federal agencies and nonfederal agencies would be expected to undertake.

4. The Target Capabilities List, which identifies areas in which responding agencies are expected to be proficient to meet the
   expectations set out in the Universal Task List.
5. The National Preparedness System sets out the framework
   through which federal agencies operate when a catastrophe
   occurs.
6. The National Incident Management System, which identifies
   standard operating procedures and approaches to be used by
   respondent agencies as they work to manage the consequences
   of a catastrophe.

According to Bea (2005), the National Preparedness System represents the most comprehensive effort taken to develop an emergency
preparedness and response system. Ultimately, the National Preparedness System is intended to increase federal involvement in emergency
preparedness and response by providing policy makers and practitioners with the ability to track and improve readiness, locate additional resources as needed, and make informed decisions regarding
risk management. The National Biosecurity Integration System is
being updated by the DHS to enhance information sharing. These up-
dates, referred to as the National Biosecurity Integration System Lite,
will integrate data from the CDC, FDA, USDA, and DHS Science Technology Directorate. National Biosecurity Integration System Lite is
intended to enable early detection and characterization of biological
trends, provide situational understanding to guide response, and enable the sharing of information among its partners. The Vulnerability Identification Self-Assessment Tool and the National Asset
Database were also developed by the DHS as a way of improving
overall preparedness (Church, 2006). The Vulnerability Identification
Self-Assessment Tool will allow a self-assessment of vulnerabilities
by various sector participants. The National Asset Database is a secure, Web-based application for the exchange of unclassified asset information and is designed to integrate with other related data
repositories. Vulnerability Identification Self-Assessment Tool assessments will be linked to the National Asset Database and will provide
a means to assess baseline security system effectiveness against a
base set of threat scenarios. Ultimately, the goal of this system is to
provide data and tools to assess and quantify risk according to the
variables of threat, vulnerability, and consequence.

The Department of Health and Human Services is the US government's principal agency for protecting the health of all Americans and providing essential human services. Eleven operating divisions, including the National Institutes of Health, the FDA, and the CDC, administer its programs. For example, the Bioterrorism Act of 2002 supplied the FDA with more authority to protect the nation's food supply against the threat of intentional contamination as well as other food-related emergencies (Food and Drug Administration, 2002; Schuchat, Aguilar, & Bender, 2005; Vogy, 2005). Section 305 of the Bioterrorism Act outlines the rules for the registration of companies involved in the food system. According to new rule, all domestic and foreign facilities that manufacture, process, pack, or hold food for human or animal consumption in the United States were required to register with the FDA no later than December 12, 2003. Registration consists of providing information, such as the firm name, address, product brands, and categories. Farms, restaurants, retail food establishments, nonprofit establishments that prepare or serve food, and fishing vessels that are not engaged in processing are exempt from this requirement.

Section 306 outlines the rules for record keeping and maintenance. This section gives the FDA authority to require that all food processors keep production and distribution records. Facilities will be required to make these records available within 24 hours in the event of a suspected food safety problem. Farmers, retailers, restaurants, and other businesses dealing directly with the public do not have to keep records; however, they are required to maintain records on where retail products were obtained.

Section 307 deals specifically with prior notice of food imports. Under the new guidelines, all food importers must give advance electronic notification to the FDA prior to the importation of food. The notice must include a description of the article, the manufacturer, the shipper, the grower, the country of origin, the country from which the article is shipped, and the anticipated port of entry.

Other issues outlined in the Bioterrorism Act include administration detention, debarment for persons convicted of conduct related to the adulteration of imported food, and allocation of grant funds to assist with the costs of enhancing food safety efforts and the costs associated with taking action when a credible threat of adulterated food is present. As mentioned previously, the overall purpose of these new guidelines is to give the FDA the authority and information needed to protect our food supply. Access to records is intended to better facilitate the tracking and control of food products suspected of being contaminated. The intended purpose of prior notification is to ensure that all imports comply with US regulations and that suspect shipments are identified and inspected. Additionally, through the use of food facility registration, the FDA will have a more accurate inventory of its regulatory domain, which will further enhance its ability to trace intentionally and unintentionally contaminated food.

> **Learning Point:** The Department of Health and Human Services is the US government's principal agency for protecting the health of all Americans and providing essential human services.

Federal responsibilities to protect the agricultural infrastructure against acts of terrorism fall primarily with the USDA. Within the USDA, the Animal and Plant Health Inspection Service (APHIS) and the Food Safety and Inspection Service (FSIS) have the primary authority to protect agriculture and ensure the safety of meat, poultry, and egg products, while the Agricultural Research Service (ARS) conducts research and development of countermeasures and diagnostic tools. Under the guidance of the USDA agencies, several important agro-security initiatives have been implemented. For example, the National Animal Identification System (NAIS), a collaborative state–federal–industry partnership, was implemented as a means to standardize and expand animal identification programs and practices to include all livestock species and poultry (USDA Animal and Plant Health Inspection Service, 2006a). The NAIS is currently being developed, under the guidance of the USDA, for all animals that will benefit from rapid tracebacks in the event of a potential disease outbreak. Many species can already be identified through some sort of identification system, but these systems are not consistently used across the United States. Under such a system, all states will operate under national standards to eliminate inconsistencies and overlap. The NAIS will integrate systems currently in place, such as premise identification, animal identification, and animal tracking systems. Eventually, it will provide health officials with the capability of identifying all livestock and premises that have had direct contact with the disease of concern within 48 hours after the discovery of a potential outbreak. The USDA hopes to make animal identification mandatory in 2008; currently, the program is voluntary.

The National Center for Animal Health Surveillance (NCAHS) was created by the USDA in 2004 as a result of the restructuring of the Center for Animal Health Monitoring (CAHM) in an effort to strengthen the US animal health surveillance system (USDA Animal and Plant Health Inspection Service, 2006b). The NCAHS is one of three centers within the Veterinary Services' Center for Epidemiology and Animal Health and is organized into two units: the National Surveillance Unit and the National Animal Health Monitoring System. The National Surveillance Unit coordinates activities related to US animal health surveillance and addresses recommendations regarding surveillance. The National Animal Health Monitoring System is responsible for collecting, analyzing, and disseminating data on animal health, management, and productivity across the United States. Information sharing was enhanced with the development of a USDA liaison position in the National Counterterrorism Center (Church, 2006). The National Counterterrorism Center was established by the president in August 2004 to serve as the primary organization in the US government for integrating and analyzing all intelligence pertaining to terrorism and counterterrorism and for conducting strategic operational planning by integrating all instruments of national power.

The USDA has also implemented several programs designed to increase education and skills among first responders. For example, the USDA is working with other federal and state agencies to outline a new education and outreach plan, which includes the development of a new Web site for bovine spongiform encephalitis information (USDA Animal and Plant Health Inspection Service, 2004).

Learning Point: The goal of USDA outreach efforts is to inform producers and affiliated industries of the surveillance goals and to encourage the reporting of suspect or targeted cattle on farms and elsewhere.

There are several examples of collaborative efforts among government agencies. For example, the Memorandum of Agreement for an Integrated Consortium of Laboratory Networks, a collaborative effort between the FDA, Centers for Disease Control and Prevention (CDC), USDA, DHS, and Environmental Protection Agency (EPA), was initiated to integrate human and animal laboratory networks (Bea, 2005). The Integrated Consortium of Laboratory Networks initially grew from the collaborative work of the US Environmental Protection Agency and the CDC and was expanded under this agreement to include other laboratory networks, such as the USDA's National Animal Health Laboratory Network and the Food Emergency Response Network, a collaborative effort between the FDA and the USDA's Food Safety and Inspection Service. The long-term goal of this collaborative effort is to provide early detection and effective consequence management of acts of terrorism and other events that involve a variety of agents or more than one segment of the nation (e.g., humans, wildlife, domestic pets, plants, food, and the environment).

The Strategic Partnership Program Agroterrorism Initiative was initiated in 2005 (Food and Drug Administration, 2005). Under this initiative, the DHS, USDA, FDA, and Federal Bureau of Investigation will collaborate with private industry and the states to help identify sectorwide vulnerabilities and develop mitigation strategies to reduce the threat of an agroterrorist attack. To facilitate the implementation of this initiative, a series of site visits at multiple food and agriculture and production facilities will be conducted to validate or identify vulnerabilities at the specific site and the sector as a whole. The information gathered from these site visits will be used to develop mitigation strategies and lessons learned. A cooperative agreement between the National Association of State Departments of Agriculture, the USDA, the FDA, and the DHS was drawn up to integrate federal and state response plans for food and agricultural emergencies (Food and Drug Administration, 2004).

Implementation of this cooperative agreement will occur in the following three phases:

1. A workgroup consisting of federal, state, and local officials will gather information about existing state emergency response systems and how food and agricultural safety and security emergencies will be handled within the various states.
2. The information gathered during phase 1, which will include state and local participation, will be used to develop an interagency response plan, to conduct tabletop exercises, to pilot test

the functionality of the emergency response plan, and to refine the plan on the basis of the lessons learned and other input.

3. The information that is gathered during phase 2 will be used to develop guidelines for federal food and agricultural regulatory agencies to cooperate with state and local emergency response efforts.

Ultimately, the goal of this initiative is to better facilitate federal assistance more quickly and appropriately to assist the local response and recovery efforts. The Food Emergency Response Plan Template is available on the National Association of State Departments of Agriculture Web site (http://www.nasda.org/cms/7196/7357/15782.aspx).

What Academic Institutions Are Doing to Improve Food Safety

Universities have taken a lead role in the area of outreach and professional development. Numerous training programs and educational Web sites have been developed to address bioterrorism education. As mentioned previously, the shortage of trained personnel in state and local public and animal health departments and laboratories is a major issue. Barriers to finding and hiring adequately trained personnel include noncompetitive salaries and a general shortage of people with the necessary skills to respond to a catastrophic event. The National Center for Food Protection and Defense, based at the University of Minnesota, was established as a Homeland Security Center of Excellence in 2004 (University of Minnesota, 2006). The National Center for Food Protection and Defense, a multidisciplinary and action-oriented consortium, addresses the issues of vulnerability to the nation's food system by:

1. making significant improvements in supply chain security, preparedness, and resiliency
2. developing rapid and accurate methods to detect incidents of contamination and to identify the specific agent(s) involved
3. applying strategies to reduce the risk of foodborne illness due to intentional contamination in the food supply chain
4. developing tools to facilitate recovery from contamination incidents and resumption of safe food system operations

5. rapidly mobilizing and delivering appropriate and credible risk communication messages to the public
6. delivering high-quality education and training programs to develop a cadre of professionals equipped to deal with future threats to the food system

The National Center for Foreign Animal and Zoonotic Disease Defense, based at Texas A&M University, was also established as a Homeland Security Center of Excellence in 2004 (Texas A&M University, 2006). Other core members of the National Center for Foreign Animal and Zoonotic Disease Defense include the University of California at Davis, the University of Southern California, and the University of Texas Medical Branch. The National Center for Foreign Animal and Zoonotic Disease Defense was designed to produce four general products:

1. specific biological research products and outcomes
2. a robust database and models that can be used to assist in making decisions, predicting needs, and testing outcomes
3. application of the models to specific needs of the department
4. expanded professional resources directed to foreign animal and zoonotic diseases, all of which are directly relevant to countering the threat of agricultural bioterrorism

The National Agricultural Biosecurity Center was established by Kansas State University in 1999 (Kansas State University, 2005). The goal of the National Agricultural Biosecurity Center is to coordinate academic agricultural biosecurity activities with federal, state, and local agencies and the public health community through the following methods:

1. response planning and exercises
2. education and awareness
3. a syndromic surveillance program
4. international initiatives
5. efforts on the part of the Biosecurity Research Institute

The Florida Department of Agriculture and Consumer Services at Florida State University has implemented the State Agricultural Response Team, which is designed to coordinate disaster response for animals and agriculture (Florida State University, 2006). The State Agricultural Response Team utilizes the skills and resources of various agencies to support the county, regional, and state emergency management efforts and incident management teams. Its mission is to provide Floridians with the necessary training and resources to enhance all-hazard disaster planning and response for animal and agricultural issues. The South Central Center for Public Health Preparedness at the University of Alabama at Birmingham, in partnership with the CDC, the Health Resources and Services Administration, and the universities and public health departments in other states, also provides public and animal health training related to agroterrorism (UAB South Central Center for Public Health Preparedness, 2005; University of Alabama at Birmingham, 2005). The South Central Center for Public Health Preparedness held its first Agricultural Security conference in June 2005. The focus of this conference was to educate public health, agricultural, regulatory, and law enforcement communities about zoonotic diseases and to foster a multiagency, multidisciplinary dialogue to ensure the safety of the food supply for all Americans. The South Central Center for Public Health Preparedness also offers several training and preparedness center courses, online courses, Webcast courses, and CD-ROMs that focus on agriculturally related issues, such as the following:

1. Improving Your Communication Skills (training course)
2. Food as an Effective Weapon of Terrorism (preparedness course)
3. The Terrorist Threat to Global Food, Water, & Agricultural Infrastructure: What Can We Do to Ensure an Ongoing & Safe Supply of Food & Water (online course)
4. Agroterrorism & Public Health—Reestablishing an Old Relationship (Webcast)
5. Emerging Infectious Diseases & Bioterrorism Risk (online course)
6. Agricultural Security—Avian Influenza: Implications for Agriculture and Public Health (Webcast, presentation from the 2005 Agricultural Security conference)
7. Bioterrorism (part 2 of the WMD [weapons of mass destruction] Terrorism Series) (CD-ROM)

To expand the pool of "first detectors," the Kentucky Injury Prevention Center at the University of Kentucky College of Public Health has collaborated with the Kentucky Department of Agriculture and the UK College of Agriculture to develop two online courses on agroterrorism education (Computer-based agroterrorism, 2005). To expand the pool of health care professionals who are able to respond to infectious disease outbreaks, the University of Alabama at Birmingham is providing online continuing education and information for rare and emerging infections and potential category A bioterrorist agents (University of Alabama at Birmingham, 2005). To help expand the veterinary workforce, the Association of American Veterinary Colleges has lobbied for support of the Veterinary Workforce Expansion Act, which has not yet been implemented (Church, 2006). The Veterinary Workforce Expansion Act is a loan repayment program for veterinarians who agree to work in "shortage situations." Such shortage situations are determined in a competitive process that is requested by state veterinarians, Area Veterinarians in Charge, and Food Safety and Inspection Service District Managers. The goal of this program is to expand capacity and services at existing schools, including teaching laboratories, research facilities, classrooms, and administrative spaces.

Several academic institutes have programs designed to increase food safety awareness among consumers. For example, Washington State University has a Web site that contains information for consumers, including food safety guidelines on topics from personal hygiene to food handling techniques (Washington State University, 2007). WSU also has an Extension Food Processing group that provides assistance and support to the food and related industries in the Northwest. The focus of this program is the safety and quality of the food supply from primary producers (growers) to the consumer, improving efficiencies within the operations, management of risks, and security of the products, facilities, and workers. They accomplish these goals through effective dissemination of information (e.g., training, seminars, workshops, and direct contacts); technology-needs identification, development, and transfer; business assessments; regulatory liaising; problem solving; and applied research. The Utah Food Safety Coalition, part of the Utah State University Extension Service, was established to enhance partnerships between government, academia, industry, and consumers through farm-to-fork food safety education programs (Utah State University Extension, 2007). Michigan State University (MSU) has several centers and programs dedicated to the enhancement of food safety (Michigan State University, 2007). For example, the Food Domain Web site, created by MSU's Voices and Visions for Food and Food Safety Project, was designed to serve as a useful food-related resource for the people of Michigan, the United States, and other countries. MSU's National Food Safety and Toxicology Center (NFSTC) was established to reduce food-related disease on a global level through research, education, and service. The Center is primarily committed to ensuring the safety of all types of food; addressing food safety-related issues in all forms and at all stages of food production; focusing efforts on the areas of greatest need; being involved in food safety activities at local, national, and international levels; and conducting activities, such as basic and applied research, in a broad range of food safety issues and food safety-related education. Iowa State University has also developed numerous programs designed to provide consumers with sources of reliable food safety information (Iowa State University, 2007b). For example, as part of the Food Safety Project, the Iowa State University Extension provides consumers with SafeFood, food safety information presented in the form of food safety lessons on their Web site. These lessons are designed to help consumers understand how knowledge about pathogen reduction, time and temperature abuse, and cleanliness will help decrease their incidence of foodborne illness. The information in these lessons is based on recommendations found in the Food Code 2005. The Food Code 2005 represents the most recent science-based information about good food safety practices. Iowa State University has also developed a Web site that provides consumers with reliable and updated food safety information. This Web site uses a database of commonly asked food safety questions that have science-based, refereed answers. This site partners with organizations and agencies nationwide that are currently providing science-based food safety information to meet three goals:

1. create and maintain a current, refereed body of answers to commonly asked food safety questions
2. recruit and retain qualified experts based on areas of expertise in food safety for answering questions
3. link consumers directly with food safety experts via a Web site

The unique aspect of this Web site is that all answers are refereed by a group of experts. Additionally, the group of experts is also available to answer consumer questions not found on the Web site. The group of experts are recruited from the following areas:

1. university researchers (e.g., faculty, extension staff, and other personnel who work in an area associated with food safety)
2. graduate students who work in and/or have experience with an area associated with food safety
3. industry representatives (i.e., people who work for companies associated with food manufacturing and processing, food service, or other areas of the food industry that impact food safety)
4. federal and state employees with a working knowledge of maintaining and improving consumer food supplies

The Food Safety Project was developed in 1995 by the Iowa State University Extension Specialists from the Departments of Food Science and Human Nutrition (FSHN); Hotel, Restaurant, and Institution Management (HRIM); and Veterinary Medicine (Iowa State University, 2006). The goal of the Food Safety Project is to develop educational materials that give the public the tools they need to minimize their risk of foodborne illness. The site is maintained by HRIM and FSHN Extension Specialists to provide food safety information to consumers, food service practitioners, and other site visitors. This site regularly receives 400,000 visitors with more than 1.2 million page views each year. The site is part of consumer and food service outreach activities in the Iowa State University Institute of Food Safety and Security. Funds for the creation and maintenance of the site were provided by a USDA grant. The Food Safety Consortium, established in 1988, consists of researchers from the University of Arkansas, Iowa State University, and Kansas State University (Iowa State University, 2007a). The consortium's charge is to conduct extensive investigation into all areas of poultry, beef, and pork meat production, from the farm to the consumer's table. Each of the university members of the consortium is primarily performing research associated with the specific animal species for which that university is uniquely qualified: University of Arkansas: poultry; Iowa State University: pork; and Kansas State University: beef. The consortium conducts research on new ways to maintain and enhance food safety by developing technology to rapidly identify contaminants, methods to evaluate potential health risks, risk-monitoring techniques to detect potential hazards in the food chain, and the most effective intervention points to control microbiological or chemical hazards.

What the Food Industry Is Doing to Improve Food Safety

The Institute of Food Technologists (IFT), founded in 1939, is a non-profit scientific society with more that 22,000 members who work in food science, food technology, and related professions in industry, academia, and government (Institute of Food Technologists, 2007). According to their Web site, IFT exists to advance the science of food, with a long-range goal of ensuring a safe and abundant food supply contributing to healthier people everywhere. To fulfill this goal, IFT focuses on the following four roles/goals:

1. providing learning, networking, and leadership development experiences that enable food science and technology professionals to become leaders in the global food science community
2. champion emerging sciences and foster technology development, application, and transfer to increase funding for food-related research and to support innovation in food science
3. engage in advocacy and communication efforts that enhance recognition of the profession and result in increased understanding and application of the science of food
4. proactively contribute to, and be a partner for, the global advancement and application of the science of food

IFT contributes to public policy and opinion at national, state, and local levels and is considered to be one of the authoritative voices of food science and technology. IFT's Office of Science, Communication, and Government Relations advocates the scientific perspective on food safety and technology issues and supports programs such as undergraduate scholarships, graduate fellowships, science-based communications to media and policy makers, career guidance programs, and food science awards. IFT also publishes various resources for the food industry, including *Food Technology* and the *Journal of Food Science*, and it conducts an annual convention on food grown, processed, manufactured, distributed, and eaten worldwide (i.e., the IFT Annual Meeting & Food Expo).

The Partnership for Food Safety Education (PFSE) is a not-for-profit organization that unites industry associations; professional societies in food science, nutrition, and health; consumer groups; and the US government to educate the public about safe food handling. PFSE is funded through contributions from industry, professional associations, consumer groups, and government agencies (Partnership for Food Safety Education, 2006). PFSE is the creator and steward of the FightBAC! campaign, a food safety initiative designed to educate consumers about the four simple practices—clean, separate, cook, and chill—that can help reduce the risk of foodborne illness. The FightBAC! campaign makes the messages accessible to everyone using the following methods:

1. Information and graphics are consumer tested, based on science, and are easy to follow.
2. They bring Americans face-to-face with the problem of foodborne illness and motivates them to take action.
3. Public opinion research and expert scientific and technical review are used to develop the messages, which reach consumers through mass media, public service announcements, the Internet, point-of-purchase, and school and community initiative.
4. A national network, which consists of public health, nutrition, food science, education, and special constituency groups, to help expand the reach of PFSE's message to all Americans.

BAC!, the campaign's "bacteria mascot," is the invisible enemy who tries to spread contamination wherever he goes. According to PFSE, giving foodborne bacteria a "personality" makes learning about the subject easier and more memorable for kids and adults. FightBAC! materials are available online, where they can be accessed by consumers, teachers, dieticians, public health officials, and extension agents across the United States.

The Food Marketing Institute (FMI) conducts programs in research, education, industry relations, and public affairs on behalf of its 1500 member companies in the United States and around the world (Food Marketing Institute, 2007). FMI's US members operate approximately 26,000 retail food stores with a combined annual sales volume of $680 billion. FMI's retail membership is composed of large multistore chains, regional firms, and independent supermarkets. Its international membership includes 200 companies from more than 50 countries. The goal of FMI is to develop and promote policies, programs, and forums that support its members, and their customers, in the following areas:

1. government relations
2. food safety and defense

3. public and consumer information
4. research and education
5. industry cooperation

FMI, which is based in Arlington, Virginia, provides a broad range of member services. FMI provides food safety programs that focus on four areas to prevent foodborne illnesses:

1. ensure that suppliers minimize contamination
2. help retailers develop science-based controls at the store level
3. train employees how to safely store, handle, and prepare foods
4. teach consumers the most basic and effective measures to safeguard products

FMI played an integral part in the development of Fight BAC! a food safety education campaign that targets consumers, students, and food retail employees. FMI is involved in food security initiatives that help educate retailers on how to protect the food supply. For example, FMI leads the Food Industry Information Sharing and Analysis Center, which works with the FBI-based National Infrastructure Protection Center to prevent and detect malicious acts to jeopardize the security of the food supply. The FMI conducts research aimed at building and maintaining a comprehensive data bank to provide members, the industry, government, and the public with well documented information, with a major emphasis placed on consumer trends, new technology, improving management practices, and total systems analysis. Additionally, FMI provides a wide range of education programs, including conferences, seminars, and training materials designed to teach skills and to improve efficiency at all levels of management. Annual conferences cover a wide range of subjects, from store security systems to food safety to recruiting, retaining, and motivating employees. The communications program provides documented, objective information about the industry performance and member views on public policy issues to the news media, government, and other interested parties. The consumer affairs program regularly liaises with consumer interest groups, serves to create an understanding of the food distributor's role in the food system, and identifies concerns of common interest among retailers and consumer representatives.

The Consulting Nutritional Services (CNS) FoodSafe, founded in 1986, provides food safety and quality assurance services in the

United States (Consulting Nutritional Services, 2007). Their customers include quick serve establishments, casual and fine dining restaurants, sports and entertainment facilities, casinos, premier hotel groups, corporate dining services, government projects, supermarkets, catering facilities, and country clubs. CNS provides food safety audits, training programs, and specialized services, such as comprehensive written reports, Web-based reporting, 24-hour foodborne illness reporting, bacterial testing, and HACCP program development.

The main goal of the CNS food safety audit program is to identify food safety and sanitation issues and provide methods to improve procedures or employee behavior to minimize risk and liability. Their auditing approach is based in the 2001 Food Code and industry-wide best practices. The audit is conducted at the time of production to see a variety of preparation and service components. At the conclusion of the audit, a written report is provided that details all areas of compliance and serves as an important tool for review and improvement. The audit report identifies priority issues that require immediate attention and noncritical issues aimed at improving food safety and food service quality. Scores for each compliance item are based on the level of importance, with more weight given to those items that are immediate risks to food safety. The final scoring provides a guideline for the overall level of compliance. The goal is to score 90% or better.

CNS offers three training programs:

1. on-site training for managers and staff
2. ServSafe Food Protection Manager Certification course
3. NSF HACCP Manager Certification Training course

The goal of the on-site training course for managers and staff is the prevention of foodborne illness. This is achieved by providing a review of good personal hygiene, implementation of time and temperature controls and proper cooling procedures, as well as many other components that follow the flow of food. The ServSafe certification course, a nationally recognized training course from the National Restaurant Association, includes testing to be ServSafe certified. The NSF HACCP training course provides certification in hazard analysis critical control points in a comprehensive, hands-on training format.

The Beef Industry Food Safety Council (BIFSCO) brings together representatives from all segments of the beef industry to develop industry-wide, science-based strategies to solve the problem of *E. coli* O157:H7 and other foodborne pathogens in beef (Beef Industry Food Safety Council, 2007). According to BIFSCO, the beef industry is challenged to recognize and address an expanding and increasingly complex food safety agenda that must serve an even more complex food delivery system. To meet these new and complex challenges, BIFSCO is striving to develop industry-wide, science-based strategies to solve the problems of foodborne pathogens in beef. To accomplish this goal, the council focuses on identifying, funding, and prioritizing research from farm-to-fork; developing programs to help industry segments operate in today's business environment; speaking with one voice in seeking regulatory and legislative solutions; developing and implementing industry information programs to assist in the transfer of technology into the marketplace; and providing pertinent, accurate, and reliable information to consumers.

The BIFSCO supports several initiatives. For example, the council supports a coordinated, proactive, industry-wide information effort for consumers. According to BIFSCO, industry should focus on all safe food handling practices in conjunction with beef-specific safety/handling information as part of that effort. In this area, the primary goals are to communicate the industry-led, farm-to-fork efforts and their results to facilitate a positive change in consumer attitudes about the safety of beef and to be a part of a campaign for consumers on their role as the "last critical control point" to change food handling/safety behaviors. Crisis communication is another priority of the council. Recent outbreaks emphasize the importance of accurate and timely information from all segments of industry. The multitude of communication points necessitates the need for a clear plan of action to prevent such outbreaks. The council supports industry informational programs. According to the council, current industry educational programs need to be expanded and coordinated to encompass a prevention-based system that can effectively meet the needs and diversity of beef-producing segments.

The US Poultry and Egg Association (PEA), formed in 1947, is the world's largest and most active poultry organization (US Poultry and Egg Association, 2007). Membership includes producers and processors of broilers, turkeys, ducks, eggs, and breeding stock, as well as allied companies. The association has affiliations in 27 states and member companies worldwide. Their mission is to partner with state affiliates and national organizations to augment and influence each other's efforts in attacking common problems. They are also committed to the advancement of research and education in poultry science and technology as well as increasing the availability and constant improvement of the quality and safety of poultry products.

Each year, PEA gives approximately $1.2 million to support research that benefits the poultry industry. The association also sponsors the International Poultry Exposition and 13 educational programs that focus on specific industry management functions. PEA maintains a multipronged communications effort to keep people in the industry current on the issues that affect their livelihoods, as well as communication efforts with the public to convey the important role the industry plays in shaping the US economy.

Chapter Summary

The nature of food and foodborne illness has changed dramatically in the United States over the past century. These changes have prompted both government and industry as well as academic institutions to initiate new strategies and collaborative efforts designed to support a comprehensive system spanning the entire food continuum. Federal agencies have implemented several programs, such as the National Biosecurity Integration System and the National Animal Identification System, that require collaboration on the part of more than one federal agency. The goal behind these new collaborative programs is to increase inspection capacity, improve surveillance, enhance response, and minimize the damage caused by a foodborne disease outbreak and other natural or manmade catastrophes.

Academic institutions and industry have taken a lead role in the development and implementation of programs designed to reduce the numbers and impact of foodborne disease outbreaks. The shortage of trained personnel in state and local public and animal health departments and laboratories continues to be a major issue. Academic institutions, such as the University of Minnesota, University of Kansas, and the University of Alabama at Birmingham, have responded to the vulnerabilities in the nation's food system by developing educational outreach programs as well as continuing the on-going efforts to develop rapid and accurate diagnostic method. Many academic institutions have implemented response planning exercises and educational awareness programs that target first responders, such as physicians, fire fighters and law enforcement, and public health workers. The goal of many of these programs is to foster multi-agency, multidisciplinary dialog. In industry, agencies such as the Institute of Food Technologists and the Partnership for Food Safety Education, provide learning, networking, and leadership development experiences for food science and technology professionals. These groups also support emerging sciences and foster innovation in food science.

Although federal agencies, academia, and industry have rallied behind this cause, much is still not known about foodborne illness. Rapid globalization of food production and trade, combined with the limited knowledge regarding foodborne pathogens and food-borne disease, has resulted in larger, less confined outbreaks. The increasing number of large outbreaks reinforces the notion that there needs to be a constant dialog between government agencies and the private sector. The programs and initiatives discussed in this chapter are a move in the right direction, but it is important that both federal agencies and the private sector take a production to consumption approach when addressing protection of the food supply. In other words, every step, from farm-to-fork, matters and should be given equal weight when planning prevention and response strategies.

Issues to Debate

1. Why do you think collaboration among governmental agencies, academia, and the private sector is so important today as opposed to 20 years ago (in terms of food safety)?
2. Do you think that the bills and directives mentioned in this chapter will help to reduce the incidence of foodborne illness in the United States? Why or why not?
3. Do you think that the collaborative efforts on the part of the government agencies will effectively reduce the number of foodborne disease outbreaks or the severity of these outbreaks? Why or why not?

4. Do you think that the contributions made by academic institutions will have a positive impact on foodborne illness? Why or why not?
5. Do you think that the efforts made by industry will have a positive impact on foodborne illness? Why or why not?

References

Bea, K. (2005). *The national preparedness system: Issues in the 109th Congress* (CRS report for Congress). Retrieved December 6, 2007, from http://fpc.state.gov

Beef Industry Food Safety Council. (2007). *What Is the Beef Industry Food Safety Council?* Retrieved December 2, 2007, from http://www.bifsco.org

Church, C. (2006). *Preparedness directorate.* Retrieved December 2, 2007, from http://executivebiz.com

Computer-based agroterrorism awareness courses. (2005). *Medical News Today.* Retrieved December 10, 2007, from http://www.medicalnewstoday.com

Consulting Nutritional Services. (2007). *CNS/Foodsafe.* Retrieved December 3, 2007, from http://www.foodsafe.com

Dyckman, L. J. (2003). *Bioterrorism: A threat to agriculture and the food supply* (Testimony before the US Senate). Retrieved December 1, 2007, from http://www.gao.gov

Federation of American Scientists. (2004). *Homeland Security Presidential Directive/HSPD-9.* Retrieved December 1, 2007, from http://www.fas.org

Florida State University. (2006). *About Florida SART. State agricultural response team.* Retrieved December 5, 2007, from http://www.flsart.org

Food and Drug Administration. (2002). *The bioterrorism act of 2002.* Retrieved December 2, 2007, from http://www.fda.gov

Food and Drug Administration. (2004). *USDA, FDA and DHS sign agreement with NASDA to make nation's agriculture and food supply more secure. US Department of Health and Human Services.* Retrieved December 6, 2007, from http://www.fda.gov

Food and Drug Administration. (2005). *Strategic partnership program agroterrorism (SPPA) initiative: A joint effort of the FBI, DHS, USDA and FDA to help secure the nation's food supply [executive summary]. Federal Bureau of Investigation.* Retrieved December 4, 2007, from http://www.cfsan.fda.gov

Food Marketing Institute. (2007). *About FMI.* Retrieved December 5, 2007, from http://www.fmi.org

Homeland Security Act. (2006). Retrieved December 1, 2007, from http://en.wikipedia.org

Institute of Food Technologists. (2007). *About IFT.* Retrieved December 5, 2007, from http://www.ift.org

Iowa State University. (2006). *About the food safety project.* Retrieved December 3, 2007, from http://www.extension.iastate.edu/foodsafety/about

Iowa State University. (2007a). *Food safety consortium.* Retrieved December 3, 2007, from http://www.foodsafety.iastate.edu

Iowa State University. (2007b). *Food safety from farm to table.* Retrieved December 5, 2007, from http://www.extension.iastate.edu

Kansas State University. (2005). *Who are we? National agricultural biosecurity center.* Retrieved December 4, 2007, from http://nabc.ksu.edu

Michigan State University. (2007). *The food domain: A comprehensive resource.* Retrieved December 16, 2007, from http://www.fooddomain.msu.edu

Nolen, R. S. (2004). *Veterinary medicine: A key component of Bush's new policy defending US agriculture from terrorism.* Retrieved December 2, 2007, from http://www.avma.org

Partnership for Food Safety Education. (2006). *About PFSE.* Retrieved December 6, 2007, from http://www.fightbac.org

Schuchat, A., Aguilar, J. R., & Bender, J. B. (2005). Compendium of measures to prevent disease associated with animals in public settings. *Morbidity and Mortality Weekly Report, 54,* 1–12.

Texas A&M University. (2006). *Welcome to the FAZD center newsroom. National center for foreign animal and zoonotic disease defense.* Retrieved December 4, 2007, from http://fazd.tamu.edu

UAB South Central Center for Public Health Preparedness. (2005). *Training professionals to protect the public.* Retrieved December 10, 2007, from http://www.southcentralpartnership.org

University of Alabama at Birmingham. (2005). *Bioterrorism and emerging infections.* Retrieved December 10, 2007, from http://www.bioterrorism.uab.edu

University of Minnesota. (2006). *Program summary. National center for food protection and defense.* Retrieved December 4, 2007, from http://www.ncfpd.umn.edu

US Department of Homeland Security. (2006). Retrieved December 1, 2007, from http://en.wikipedia.org

US Poultry and Egg Association. (2007). *About us.* Retrieved December 7, 2007, from http://www.poultryegg.org

USDA Animal and Plant Health Inspection Service. (2004). *BSE update. US Department of Agriculture, Animal and Plant Health Inspection Service.* Retrieved December 2, 2007, from http://www.aphis.usda.gov

USDA Animal and Plant Health Inspection Service. (2006a). *National animal identification system. US Department of Agriculture, Animal and Plant Health Inspection Service.* Retrieved December 2, 2007, from http://animalid.aphis.usda.gov/nais/

USDA Animal and Plant Health Inspection Service. (2006b). *Animal health monitoring and surveillance. US Department of Agriculture, Animal and Plant Health Inspection Service.* Retrieved December 3, 2007, from http://www.aphis.usda.gov

Utah State University Extension. (2007). *Food safety.* Retrieved December 3, 2007, from http://extension.usu.edu

Vogy, D. U. (2005). *Food safety issues in the 109th Congress* (CRS report for Congress). Retrieved December 3, 2007, from http://italy.usembassy.gov

Washington State University. (2007). *Information for consumers.* Retrieved December 16, 2007, from http://foodsafety.wsu.edu

White House. (2003). *Homeland Security Presidential Directive/HSPD-7.* Retrieved December 1, 2007, from http://www.whitehouse.gov

INDEX